Complementary and Alternative Medicine Information for Teens

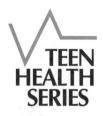

TEEN
HEALTH
SERIES

First Edition

Complementary and Alternative Medicine Information for Teens

Health Tips about Non-Traditional and Non-Western Medical Practices

Including Information about Acupuncture, Chiropractic Medicine, Dietary and Herbal Supplements, Hypnosis, Massage Therapy, Prayer and Spirituality, Reflexology, Yoga, and More

◆

Edited by Sandra Augustyn Lawton

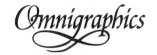

Omnigraphics

615 Griswold Street • Detroit, MI 48226

Bibliographic Note

Because this page cannot legibly accommodate all the copyright notices, the Bibliographic Note portion of the Preface constitutes an extension of the copyright notice.

Edited by Sandra Augustyn Lawton

Teen Health Series

Karen Bellenir, *Managing Editor*
David A. Cooke, M.D., *Medical Consultant*
Elizabeth Collins, *Research and Permissions Coordinator*
Cherry Stockdale, *Permissions Assistant*
Laura Pleva Nielsen, *Index Editor*
EdIndex, Services for Publishers, *Indexers*

* * *

Omnigraphics, Inc.

Matthew P. Barbour, *Senior Vice President*
Kay Gill, *Vice President—Directories*
Kevin Hayes, *Operations Manager*
David P. Bianco, *Marketing Director*

* * *

Peter E. Ruffner, *Publisher*
Frederick G. Ruffner, Jr., *Chairman*
Copyright © 2007 Omnigraphics, Inc.
ISBN 0-7808-0966-1

Library of Congress Cataloging-in-Publication Data

Complementary and alternative medicine information for teens : health tips about non-traditional and non-western medical practices including information about acupuncture, chiropractic medicine, dietary and herbal supplements, hypnosis, massage therapy, prayer and spirituality, reflexology, yoga, and more / edited by Sandra Augustyn Lawton.
    p. cm. -- (Teen health series)
    Summary: "Provides basic consumer health information for teens on non-traditional medicine and therapies. Includes index and resource information"--Provided by publisher.
    Includes bibliographical references and index.
    ISBN 0-7808-0966-1 (hardcover : alk. paper) 1. Alternative medicine--Popular works. 2. Teenagers--Health and hygiene--Popular works.
    I. Lawton, Sandra Augustyn.
    R733.C6556 2006
    610--dc22
                                                                    2006027704

Table of Contents

Preface ix

Part I: An Introduction To Complementary And Alternative Medicine

Chapter 1—What Is Complementary And Alternative Medicine? 3

Chapter 2—The Use Of Complementary And Alternative
Medicine In The United States 7

Chapter 3—Are You Considering Using Complementary
And Alternative Medicine? 13

Chapter 4—Selecting A Practitioner For Complementary
And Alternative Medical Care 23

Part II: Whole Medical Systems

Chapter 5—Whole Medical Systems: An Overview 31

Chapter 6—Ayurvedic Medicine 39

Chapter 7—Homeopathy 51

Chapter 8—Naturopathic Medicine 59

Chapter 9—Osteopathic Medicine 67

Chapter 10—Traditional Chinese Medicine 71

Chapter 11—Traditional Native American Medicine 79

Part III: Manipulative And Body-Based Practices

Chapter 12—Manipulative And Body-Based Practices:
An Overview 85

Chapter 13—Acupressure 91

Chapter 14—Acupuncture 95

Chapter 15—Alexander Technique 101

Chapter 16—Applied Kinesiology 105

Chapter 17—Chiropractic Medicine 111

Chapter 18—Craniosacral Therapy 121

Chapter 19—Hydrotherapy 125

Chapter 20—Massage Therapy 131

Chapter 21—Reflexology 135

Chapter 22—Rolfing 139

Part IV: Dietary And Herbal Remedies

Chapter 23—Dietary Supplements 145

Chapter 24—Botanical Supplements 157

Chapter 25—Detox Diets 165

Chapter 26—Macrobiotic Diet 169

Chapter 27—Raw Food Diet 173

Chapter 28—Vegetarian Diets 177

Part V: Mind-Body Medicine

Chapter 29—Mind-Body Medicine: An Overview 185

Chapter 30—Biofeedback 191

Chapter 31—Guided Imagery And Visualization 195

Chapter 32—Hypnosis 201

Chapter 33—Meditation 207

Chapter 34—Prayer And Spirituality 215

Chapter 35—Qigong 219

Chapter 36—Tai Chi 223

Chapter 37—Yoga 227

Part VI: Biologically Based Practices And Energy Medicine

Chapter 38—Apitherapy 235

Chapter 39—Chelation Therapy 239

Chapter 40—Crystal And Gemstone Therapy 243

Chapter 41—Enzyme Therapy 249

Chapter 42—Probiotics 255

Chapter 43—Magnetic Therapy 263

Chapter 44—Reiki 269

Chapter 45—Therapeutic Touch 277

Part VII: Using The Senses And Emotions To Enhance Well-Being

Chapter 46—Aromatherapy 285

Chapter 47—Art Therapy 289

Chapter 48—Dance Therapy 293

Chapter 49—Humor Therapy 297

Chapter 50—Light Therapy 301

Chapter 51—Music Therapy 311

Part VIII: Alternative Treatments For Specific Diseases And Conditions

Chapter 52—Pain Management Using Complementary
And Alternative Methods 317

Chapter 53—Cancer And Complementary And
Alternative Medicine 329

Chapter 54—Diabetes And Complementary And
Alternative Medicine 337

Chapter 55—Mental Health And Alternative Approaches 341

Part IX: If You Need More Information

Chapter 56—Getting Health Information From
Trusted Sources 349

Chapter 57—Fraudulent Health Claims: Don't Be Fooled 353

Chapter 58—How To Find Out If Your Insurance
Covers CAM Treatments 365

Chapter 59—Additional Reading About Complementary
And Alternative Medicine 375

Chapter 60—Complementary And Alternative Medicine:
A Directory Of Resources 383

Index 393

Preface

About This Book

Complementary and alternative medicine (CAM) comprises a group of health care systems, practices, and products that differ from those employed by conventional Western medicine. The term "complementary" refers to the use of such practices together with conventional medicine; "alternative" refers to their use in place of conventional medicine. People turn to CAM for various reasons. Many who use it in combination with conventional medicine seek added benefits from it—either to improve their condition or to mitigate the side effects of standard treatments. Others turn to it because they perceive it as a natural way to treat or avoid illness. For some, it is a last resort.

Complementary And Alternative Medicine Information For Teens provides information about whole medical systems that developed independently from Western medical theories, including traditional Chinese medicine, ayurvedic (traditional Indian/Hindu) medicine, traditional Native American medicine, homeopathy, and naturopathic medicine. It also describes commonly used practices and therapies, such as chiropractic adjustment, massage therapy, dietary and herbal remedies, hypnosis, meditation, and aromatherapy. A separate section discusses the use of CAM therapies in the treatment of cancer, diabetes, chronic pain, and mental illness—disorders that often present special challenges to conventional medicine. The text concludes with suggestions for additional reading and a directory of resources.

How To Use This Book

This book is divided into parts and chapters. Parts focus on broad areas of interest; chapters are devoted to single topics within a part.

Part I: An Introduction To Complementary And Alternative Medicine describes CAM, who uses it, and why. Guidelines for selecting CAM methods and practitioners are also included.

Part II: Whole Medical Systems discusses wellness theories and healing practices that evolved separately from, or parallel to, Western medicine. Whole medical systems include ayurvedic medicine, homeopathy, naturopathic medicine, traditional Chinese medicine, and traditional Native American medicine.

Part III: Manipulative And Body-Based Practices provides facts about the various interventions and therapies that focus primarily on the structures and systems of the body. These include acupressure, acupuncture, Alexander technique, applied kinesiology, chiropractic medicine, craniosacral therapy, hydrotherapy, massage therapy, reflexology, and Rolfing.

Part IV: Dietary And Herbal Remedies describes the use of dietary and botanical supplements as health aides. It also discusses several specific diets that people sometimes adopt for medical reasons.

Part V: Mind-Body Medicine presents information on using the power of thoughts and emotions to positively influence physical health. These therapies include biofeedback, guided imagery and visualization, hypnosis, meditation, prayer and spirituality, qigong, tai chi, and yoga.

Part VI: Biologically Based Practices And Energy Medicine discusses techniques that seek to enhance biological processes and manipulate body energy. These include apitherapy, chelation therapy, crystal and gemstone therapy, enzyme therapy, probiotics, magnetic therapy, Reiki, and therapeutic touch.

Part VII: Using The Senses And Emotions To Enhance Well-Being explains how some therapies use the senses and emotions to enhance an individual's wellbeing. Included in this group are aromatherapy, light therapy, humor therapy, and art, dance, and music therapy.

Part VIII: Alternative Treatments For Specific Diseases And Conditions discusses how CAM methods are used to manage pain, treat cancer and diabetes, and address mental health issues.

Part IX: If You Need More Information provides guidelines for students who would like to pursue additional research about CAM practices. It explains how to assess health claims and discusses the limitations traditional health insurance policies often place on CAM therapies. The part concludes with suggestions for further reading and a directory of CAM resources.

Bibliographic Note

This volume contains documents and excerpts from publications issued by the following government agencies: Indian Health Service; National Cancer Institute (NCI); National Center for Complementary and Alternative Medicine (NCCAM); National Diabetes Information Clearinghouse (NDIC); National Women's Health Information Center (NWHIC); Office of Dietary Supplements; Substance Abuse and Mental Health Services Administration (SAMHSA); U.S. Department of Agriculture; U.S. Department of Labor; U.S. Federal Trade Commission; and the U.S. Food and Drug Administration.

In addition, this volume contains copyrighted documents and articles produced by the following organizations and individuals: About, Inc.; A.D.A.M., Inc.; American Apitherapy Society; American Art Therapy Association; American Association of Colleges of Osteopathic Medicine; American Association of Naturopathic Physicians; American Dance Therapy Association; American Heart Association; American Medical Student Association; American Music Therapy Association; American Society of Clinical Hypnosis; Association of Cancer Online Resources; Association of Reflexologists; Better Health Channel (Victoria, Australia); California Dairy Research Foundation; Creighton University School of Medicine; Virginia Evangelou; Gale Group; International Center for Reiki Training; International College of Applied Kinesiology; Medical College of Georgia; National Qigong Association; Nemours Foundation; Rolf Institute; Society for Light Treatment and Biological Rhythms; Upledger Institute; and Whole Health Chicago.

The collection of documents reprinted in this book describes CAM practices, and it comments on how to evaluate whether or not they are effective. Some individual documents were written by CAM practitioners and advocates; others were written by organizations holding a more skeptical point of view.

Taken as a whole, this diversity of opinion helps explain multifaceted, and often controversial, issues. Individually, however, each of the various documents that comprise the chapters of this book presents information from a particular point of view. Readers can be better informed about the potential bias of specific information by noting its producer. To help assist in that process, full citation information for the text in each chapter is provided on the chapter's first page. When supplemented facts, tips, or explanatory notes appearing in sidebars are from other sources, the sidebars carry additional citations.

The photograph on the front cover is from mandygodbehear/istock.com.

Every effort has been made to secure all necessary rights to reprint the copyrighted material. If any omissions have been made, please contact Omnigraphics to make corrections for future editions.

Acknowledgements

In addition to the organizations listed above, special thanks are due to research and permissions coordinator Elizabeth Collins and to managing editor Karen Bellenir.

About the *Teen Health Series*

At the request of librarians serving today's young adults, the *Teen Health Series* was developed as a specially focused set of volumes within Omnigraphics' *Health Reference Series*. Each volume deals comprehensively with a topic selected according to the needs and interests of people in middle school and high school.

Teens seeking preventive guidance, information about disease warning signs, medical statistics, and risk factors for health problems will find answers to their questions in the *Teen Health Series*. The *Series*, however, is not intended to serve as a tool for diagnosing illness, in prescribing treatments, or as a substitute for the physician/patient relationship. All people concerned about medical symptoms or the possibility of disease are encouraged to seek professional care from an appropriate health care provider.

If there is a topic you would like to see addressed in a future volume of the *Teen Health Series*, please write to:

Editor, *Teen Health Series*
Omnigraphics, Inc.
615 Griswold Street
Detroit, MI 48226

Locating Information within the *Teen Health Series*

The *Teen Health Series* contains a wealth of information about a wide variety of medical topics. As the *Series* continues to grow in size and scope, locating the precise information needed by a specific student may become more challenging. To address this concern, information about books within the *Teen Health Series* is included in *A Contents Guide to the Health Reference Series*. The *Contents Guide* presents an extensive list of more than 12,000 diseases, treatments, and other topics of general interest compiled from the Tables of Contents and major index headings from the books of the *Teen Health Series* and *Health Reference Series*. To access *A Contents Guide to the Health Reference Series*, visit www.healthreferenceseries.com.

Our Advisory Board

We would like to thank the following advisory board members for providing guidance to the development of this *Series*:

Dr. Lynda Baker, Associate Professor of Library and Information Science, Wayne State University, Detroit, MI

Nancy Bulgarelli, William Beaumont Hospital Library, Royal Oak, MI

Karen Imarisio, Bloomfield Township Public Library, Bloomfield Township, MI

Karen Morgan, Mardigian Library, University of Michigan-Dearborn, Dearborn, MI

Rosemary Orlando, St. Clair Shores Public Library, St. Clair Shores, MI

Medical Consultant

Medical consultation services are provided to the *Teen Health Series* editors by David A. Cooke, M.D. Dr. Cooke is a graduate of Brandeis University, and he received his M.D. degree from the University of Michigan. He completed residency training at the University of Wisconsin Hospital and Clinics. He is board-certified in internal medicine. Dr. Cooke currently works as part of the University of Michigan Health System and practices in Ann Arbor, MI. In his free time, he enjoys writing, science fiction, and spending time with his family.

Part One
An Introduction To Complementary And Alternative Medicine

Chapter 1

What Is Complementary And Alternative Medicine?

Complementary and alternative medicine (CAM) is a group of diverse medical and health care systems, practices, and products that are not presently considered to be part of conventional medicine. While some scientific evidence exists regarding some CAM therapies, for most there are key questions that are yet to be answered through well-designed scientific studies—questions such as whether these therapies are safe and whether they work for the diseases or medical conditions for which they are used.

Are complementary medicine and alternative medicine different from each other?

Yes, they are different.

Complementary medicine is used **together with** conventional medicine. An example of a complementary therapy is using aromatherapy to help lessen a patient's discomfort following surgery.

Alternative medicine is used **in place of** conventional medicine. An example of an alternative therapy is using a special diet to treat cancer instead

About This Chapter: Information in this chapter is excerpted from "What Is Complementary and Alternative Medicine (CAM)," National Center for Complementary and Alternative Medicine (NCCAM), National Institutes of Health, NCCAM Publication No. D156, May 2002.

of undergoing surgery, radiation, or chemo-therapy that has been recommended by a conventional doctor.

What is integrative medicine?

Integrative medicine combines mainstream medical therapies and CAM therapies for which there is some high-quality scientific evidence of safety and effectiveness.

♣ **It's A Fact!!**
The list of what is considered to be complementary and alternative medicine changes continually, as those therapies that are proven to be safe and effective become adopted into conventional health care and as new approaches to health care emerge.

What are the major types of complementary and alternative medicine?

- **Alternative (or Whole) Medical Systems:** Alternative (or whole) medical systems are built upon complete systems of theory and practice. Often, these systems have evolved apart from and earlier than the conventional medical approach used in the United States. Examples of alternative medical systems that have developed in Western cultures include homeopathic medicine and naturopathic medicine. Examples of systems that have developed in non-Western cultures include traditional Chinese medicine and Ayurveda.

- **Mind-Body Interventions:** Mind-body medicine uses a variety of techniques designed to enhance the mind's capacity to affect bodily function and symptoms. Some techniques that were considered CAM in the past have become mainstream (for example, patient support groups and cognitive-behavioral therapy). Other mind-body techniques are still considered CAM, including meditation, prayer, mental healing, and therapies that use creative outlets such as art, music, or dance.

- **Biologically Based Therapies:** Biologically based therapies in CAM use substances found in nature, such as herbs, foods, and vitamins. Some examples include dietary supplements, herbal products, and the use of other so-called natural but as yet scientifically unproven therapies (for example, using shark cartilage to treat cancer).

- **Manipulative and Body-Based Methods:** Manipulative and body-based methods in CAM are based on manipulation and/or movement of one or more parts of the body. Two examples include chiropractic manipulation and massage.

- **Energy Therapies:** Energy therapies involve the use of energy fields. They are of two types:

  - **Biofield therapies** are intended to affect energy fields that purportedly surround and penetrate the human body. The existence of such fields has not yet been scientifically proven. Some forms of energy therapy manipulate biofields by applying pressure and/or manipulating the body by placing the hands in, or through, these fields. Examples include qigong, Reiki, and therapeutic touch.

  - **Bioelectromagnetic-based therapies** involve the unconventional use of electromagnetic fields, such as pulsed fields, magnetic fields, or alternating current or direct current fields.

Chapter 2

The Use Of Complementary And Alternative Medicine In The United States

Americans are using complementary and alternative medicine (CAM). But, it is often asked, how many Americans? What therapies are they using? For what health problems and concerns?

The most comprehensive and reliable findings to date on Americans' use of CAM were released in May 2004 by the National Center for Complementary and Alternative Medicine (NCCAM) and the National Center for Health Statistics (NCHS, part of the Centers for Disease Control and Prevention). They came from the 2002 edition of the NCHS's National Health Interview Survey (NHIS), an annual study in which tens of thousands of Americans are interviewed about their health- and illness-related experiences. The 2002 edition included detailed questions on CAM. It was completed by 31,044 adults aged 18 years or older from the U.S. civilian noninstitutionalized population.

CAM Therapies Included In The Survey

The survey included questions on various types of CAM therapies commonly used in the United States. These included provider-based therapies,

About This Chapter: Information in this chapter is excerpted from "The Use of Complementary and Alternative Medicine in the United States," National Center for Complementary and Alternative Medicine (NCCAM), National Institutes of Health, September 2004.

such as acupuncture and chiropractic, and other therapies that do not require a provider, such as natural products, special diets, and megavitamin
therapy. The complete list of therapies that were included in the survey is
as follows:

- Acupuncture*
- Ayurveda*
- Biofeedback*
- Chelation therapy*
- Chiropractic care*
- Deep breathing exercises
- Diet-based therapies

    Atkins diet

    Macrobiotic diet

    Ornish diet

    Pritikin diet

    Vegetarian diet

    Zone diet

- Energy healing therapy*
- Folk medicine*
- Guided imagery
- Homeopathic treatment
- Hypnosis*
- Massage*
- Meditation
- Megavitamin therapy
- Natural products

    (nonvitamin and nonmineral, such as herbs and other products
    from plants, enzymes, etc.)

- Naturopathy*

- Prayer for health reasons
    Healing ritual for self
    Others ever prayed for your health
    Participate in prayer group
    Prayed for own health
- Progressive relaxation
- Qigong
- Reiki*
- Tai chi
- Yoga

An asterisk (*) indicates a practitioner-based therapy.

The results were analyzed including and excluding two therapies—prayer specifically for health reasons and megavitamins—because earlier national surveys did not consistently include these therapies.

Unless noted otherwise, the statistics are for CAM use during the 12 months prior to the 2002 survey.

Percentage Of People Who Use CAM

In the United States, 36% of adults are using some form of CAM. When megavitamin therapy and prayer specifically for health reasons are included in the definition of CAM, that number rises to 62%.

People Who Use CAM The Most

CAM use spans people of all backgrounds; but according to the survey, some people are more likely than others to use CAM. Overall, CAM use is greater by:

- women than men;
- people with higher educational levels;
- people who have been hospitalized in the past year; and
- former smokers, compared with current smokers or those who have never smoked.

CAM Domains Used The Most

When prayer is included in the definition of CAM, the domain of mind-body medicine is the most commonly used domain (53%). (See Figure 2.1.) When prayer is not included, biologically based therapies (22%) are more popular than mind-body medicine (17%).

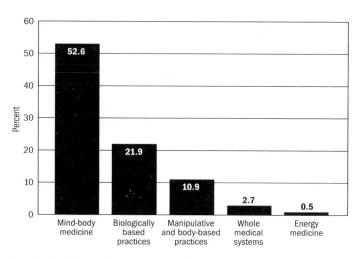

Figure 2.1. CAM Use by Domain and Whole Medical Systems

CAM Therapies Used The Most

Prayer specifically for health reasons was the most commonly used CAM therapy. (See Figure 2.2, which shows the percentage of people using each of the 10 most common therapies.) Most people who use CAM use it to treat themselves, as only about 12% of the survey respondents sought care from a licensed CAM practitioner.

Health Conditions Prompting CAM Use

People use CAM for a wide array of diseases and conditions. According to the survey, Americans are most likely to use CAM for back, neck, head, joint aches, or other painful conditions, colds, anxiety or depression, gastrointestinal disorders, or sleeping problems. (See Figure 2.3.) It appears that CAM is most often used to treat and/or prevent musculoskeletal conditions or other conditions involving chronic or recurring pain.

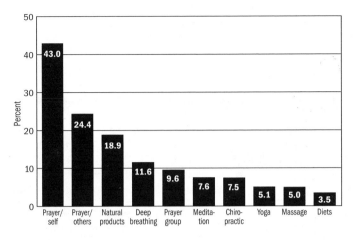

Figure 2.2. Ten Most Common CAM Therapies

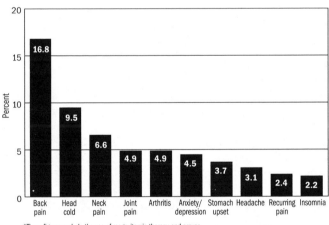

*These figures exclude the use of megavitamin therapy and prayer.

Figure 2.3. Disease/Condition for Which CAM Is Most Frequently Used

Reasons For Using CAM

The survey asked people to select from five reasons to describe why they used CAM. Results were as follows (people could select more than one reason):

- CAM would improve health when used in combination with conventional medical treatments: 55%.

- CAM would be interesting to try: 50%.

- Conventional medical treatments would not help: 28%.

- A conventional medical professional suggested trying CAM: 26%.

- Conventional medical treatments are too expensive: 13%.

The survey found that most people use CAM along with conventional medicine rather than in place of conventional medicine.

Spending On CAM

The NHIS did not include questions on spending on health care, but the report authors cited spending figures from national surveys conducted in 1997. Those surveys revealed the following information:

- The U.S. public spent an estimated $36 billion to $47 billion on CAM therapies in 1997.

- Of this amount, between $12 billion and $20 billion was paid out-of-pocket for the services of professional CAM health care providers.

- These fees represented more than the public paid out-of-pocket for all hospitalizations in 1997 and about half of what it paid for all out-of-pocket physician services.

- $5 billion of out-of-pocket spending was on herbal products.

Chapter 3

Are You Considering Using Complementary And Alternative Medicine?

Decisions about your health care are important, including decisions about whether to use complementary and alternative medicine (CAM). This chapter will assist you in your decision making about CAM. It includes frequently asked questions and issues to consider.

How can I get reliable information about a CAM therapy?

It is important to learn what scientific studies have discovered about the therapy in which you are interested. It is not a good idea to use a CAM therapy simply because of something you have seen in an advertisement or on a website or because someone has told you that it worked for them. Understanding a treatment's risks, potential benefits, and scientific evidence is critical to your health and safety. Scientific research on many CAM therapies is relatively new, so this kind of information may not be available for every therapy. However, many studies on CAM treatments are under way. Here are some ways to find scientifically based information:

- Talk to your health care practitioner(s). Tell them about the therapy you are considering and ask any questions you may have about safety,

About This Chapter: Information in this chapter is excerpted from "Are You Considering Using Complementary and Alternative Medicine (CAM)?" National Center for Complementary and Alternative Medicine (NCCAM), National Institutes of Health, NCCAM Publication No. D167, August 2002.

effectiveness, or interactions with medications (prescription or non-prescription). They may know about the therapy and be able to advise you on its safety and use. If your practitioner cannot answer your questions, he may be able to refer you to someone who can. Your practitioner may also be able to help you interpret the results of scientific articles you have found.

• Use the internet to search medical libraries and databases for information.

• Visit your local library or a medical library to see if there are books or publications that contain scientific articles discussing CAM in general or the treatment in which you are interested. Thousands of articles on health issues and CAM are published in books and scientific journals every year. A reference librarian can help you search for those on the therapy that interests you.

✔ Quick Tip
What questions should be asked when evaluating website information?

• Who runs the site? Is it government, a university, or a reputable medical or health-related association? Is it sponsored by a manufacturer of products, drugs, etc.? It should be easy to identify the sponsor.

• What is the purpose of the site? Is it to educate the public or to sell a product? The purpose should be clearly stated.

• What is the basis of the information? Is it based on scientific evidence with clear references? Advice and opinions should be clearly set apart from the science.

• How current is the information? Is it reviewed and updated frequently?

Source: Excerpted from "Are You Considering Using Complementary and Alternative Medicine (CAM)?" National Center for Complementary and Alternative Medicine (NCCAM), National Institutes of Health, NCCAM Publication No. D167, August 2002.

Are CAM therapies safe?

Each treatment needs to be considered on its own. However, here are some issues to think about when considering a CAM therapy:

- Many consumers believe that "natural" means the same thing as "safe." This is not necessarily true. For example, think of mushrooms that grow in the wild; some are safe to eat, while others are poisonous.

- Individuals respond differently to treatments. How a person might respond to a CAM treatment depends on many things, including the person's state of health, how the treatment is used, or the person's belief in the treatment.

- For a CAM product that is sold over the counter (without a prescription), such as a dietary supplement, safety can also depend on a number of things:

    - The components or ingredients that make up the product

    - Where the components or ingredients come from

    - The quality of the manufacturing process (for example, how well the manufacturer is able to avoid contamination)

- The manufacturer of a dietary supplement is responsible for ensuring the safety and effectiveness of the product before it is sold. The U.S. Food and Drug Administration (FDA) cannot require testing of dietary supplements prior to marketing. However, while manufacturers are prohibited from selling dangerous products, the FDA can remove a product from the marketplace if the product is dangerous to the health of Americans. Furthermore, if in the labeling or marketing of a dietary supplement a claim is made that the product can diagnose, treat, cure, or prevent disease, such as "cures cancer," the product is said to be an unapproved new drug and is, therefore, being sold illegally. Such claims must have scientific proof.

- For CAM therapies that are administered by a practitioner, the training, skill, and experience of the practitioner affect safety. However, in spite of careful and skilled practice, all treatments, whether CAM or conventional, can have risks.

How can I determine whether statements made about the effectiveness of a CAM therapy are true?

Statements that manufacturers and providers of CAM therapies may make about the effectiveness of a therapy and its other benefits can sound reasonable and promising. However, they may or may not be backed up by scientific evidence. Before you begin using a CAM treatment, it is a good idea to ask the following questions:

- Is there scientific evidence (not just personal stories) to back up the statements? Ask the manufacturer or the practitioner for scientific articles or the results of studies. They should be willing to share this information, if it exists.

- Does the federal government have anything to report about the therapy?

  - Visit the FDA online at www.fda.gov to see if there is any information available about the product or practice. Information specifically about dietary supplements can be found on FDA's Center for Food Safety and Applied Nutrition website at www.cfsan.fda.gov or visit the FDA's web page on recalls and safety alerts at www.fda.gov/opacom/7alerts.html.

  - Check with the Federal Trade Commission (FTC) at www.ftc.gov to see if there are any fraudulent claims or consumer alerts regarding the therapy. Visit the Diet, Health, and Fitness Consumer Information website at www.ftc.gov/bcp/menu-health.htm.

  - Visit the National Center for Complementary and Alternative Medicine (NCCAM) website, http://nccam.nih.gov, or call the NCCAM Clearinghouse to see if NCCAM has any information or scientific findings to report about the therapy.

- How does the provider or manufacturer describe the treatment? The FDA advises that certain types of language may sound impressive but actually disguise a lack of science. Be wary of terminology such as "innovation," "quick cure," "miracle cure," "exclusive product," "new discovery," or "magical discovery." Watch out for claims of a "secret formula." If a therapy were a cure for a disease, it would be widely reported and prescribed or recommended. Legitimate scientists want to share their knowledge so that their peers can review their data. Be suspicious of phrases like "suppressed by government" or claims that the medical profession or research scientists have conspired to prevent a therapy from reaching the public. Finally, be wary of claims that something cures a wide range of unrelated diseases (for example, cancer, diabetes, and AIDS). No product can treat every disease and condition.

Are there any risks to using CAM treatments?

Yes, there can be risks, as with any medical therapy. These risks depend upon the specific CAM treatment. The following are general suggestions to help you learn about or minimize the risks:

- Discuss with your health care practitioner any CAM treatment that you are considering or are using; it is important for your safety and for a comprehensive treatment plan. For example, herbal or botanical products and other dietary supplements may interact with medications (prescription or non-prescription). They may also have negative, even dangerous, effects on their own. Research has shown that the herb St. John's wort, which is used by some people to treat depression, may cause certain drugs to become less effective. And kava, an herb that has been used for insomnia, stress, and anxiety, has been linked to liver damage.

- If you have more than one health care provider, let all of them know about CAM and conventional therapies you are using. This will help each provider make sure that all aspects of your health care work together.

- Take charge of your health by being an informed consumer. Find out what the scientific evidence is about any treatment's safety and whether it works.

- If you decide to use a CAM treatment that would be given by a practitioner, choose the practitioner carefully to help minimize any possible risks.

✔ Quick Tip

How should I talk to my doctor about alternative medicines?

The popularity of complementary and alternative medicine is on the rise, with more than one-third of U.S. adults using at least one of these treatments, according to a recent report by the Institute of Medicine.

If you're like most proponents of these treatments, you probably don't mention them to your primary-care physician. You may think it's not important, you might just forget or you might think your doctor won't approve.

But it's crucial to tell your doctor, says Dr. Robert Bonakdar, a family physician at the Scripps Center for Integrative Medicine in La Jolla, California who directs pain management and blends conventional and alternative approaches.

"Everything a patient is using is important for the doctor to know," he says. "Full disclosure enables full care."

Another physician with a special interest in integrative medicine agrees. "The best thing patients can do is be honest with what they are taking," says Dr. Janine Blackman, medical director of The Center for Integrative Medicine at the University of Maryland, Baltimore and an assistant professor of family medicine.

Complementary and alternative medicine describes a wide group of medical practices and products, according to the National Institutes of Health's National Center for Complementary and Alternative Medicine. Complementary describes techniques used in conjunction with conventional medicine; alternative describes techniques that can be used in place of it.

Among the options are homeopathic medicine, chiropractic, dietary supplements, aromatherapy, and massage therapy, among many others.

so, how best to approach your doctor? First, understand that your doctor may not have a lot of background or knowledge about an alternative or complementary approach, Bonakdar says. Few doctors, especially older ones, studied these treatments in medical school.

"Bring it up in an open manner," he suggests, by saying something like, "This is something I am interested in, what do you think?"

Physicians should be open to discussion, at least, he says. "The patients should expect the doctor to be open and non-judgmental in the discussion of complementary treatments," he said. "They should hear you out."

"They should be able to educate you from their standpoint based on whether they think it is safe, appropriate and effective," he adds. As a patient, you should expect your physician, if he or she is unfamiliar with the treatment you are interested in, to offer to check to see if there is any evidence that it works, Bonakdar says.

In recent years, Blackman adds, more physicians have become open to the concept of alternative medicine or complementary approaches.

But a recent survey, published in the Archives of Internal Medicine, found that 84 percent of the 302 physicians questioned thought they needed to know more about complementary and alternative medicine to address patient questions and concerns adequately. Even so, nearly half had recommended an alternative or complementary treatment to a patient.

One way to facilitate the discussion about alternative or complementary treatments is to bring as much information as you can to the doctor visit. If you're interested in supplements, for instance, take the bottle so the doctor can see the exact dose and formula, plus the manufacturer.

Patients must understand there are dangers to mixing some complementary and conventional treatments, Blackman says. Certain dietary supplements, for instance, can affect the dosing of blood-thinning medications, thinning the blood to adverse levels, she says.

If your doctor isn't comfortable with an alternative or complementary approach that you feel strongly about, you have options, Blackman maintains. Either find a new physician or continue seeing your doctor, alerting him or her about your decision to use the complementary or alternative approach. Then, you can consult someone else knowledgeable about the alternative therapy, such as a pharmacist.

Are CAM therapies tested to see if they work?

While some scientific evidence exists regarding the effectiveness of some CAM therapies, for most there are key questions that are yet to be answered through well-designed scientific studies—questions such as whether they are safe, how they work, and whether they work for the diseases or medical conditions for which they are used.

NCCAM is the federal government's lead agency on scientific research of CAM. NCCAM supports research on CAM therapies to determine if they work, how they work, whether they are effective, and who might benefit most from the use of specific therapies.

I am interested in a CAM therapy that involves treatment from a practitioner. How do I go about selecting a practitioner?

Here are a few things to consider when selecting a practitioner.

- Ask your physician, other health professionals, or someone you believe to be knowledgeable regarding CAM whether they have recommendations.

- Contact a nearby hospital or a medical school and ask if they maintain a list of area CAM practitioners or could make a recommendation. Some regional medical centers may have a CAM center or CAM practitioners on staff.

- Contact a professional organization for the type of practitioner you are seeking. Often, professional organizations have standards of practice, provide referrals to practitioners, have publications explaining the therapy (or therapies) that their members provide, and may offer information on the type of training needed and whether practitioners of a therapy must be licensed or certified in your state. Professional organizations can be located by searching the internet or directories in libraries (ask the librarian). One directory is the Directory of Information Resources Online (DIRLINE) compiled by the National Library of Medicine (http://dirline.nlm.nih.gov). It contains locations and descriptive information about a variety of health organizations, including CAM associations and organizations.

- Many states have regulatory agencies or licensing boards for certain types of practitioners. They may be able to provide you with information regarding practitioners in your area. Your state, county, or city health department may be able to refer you to such agencies or boards. Licensing, accreditation, and regulatory laws for CAM practices are becoming more common to help ensure that practitioners are competent and provide quality services.

Chapter 4

Selecting A Practitioner For Complementary And Alternative Medical Care

Selecting a health care practitioner of conventional or complementary and alternative medicine (CAM) is an important decision and can be key to ensuring that you are receiving the best health care. This chapter will answer frequently asked questions about selecting a CAM practitioner, such as issues to consider when making your decision and important questions to ask the practitioner you select.

I am interested in a CAM therapy that involves treatment from a practitioner. How do I go about finding a practitioner?

Here are some suggestions for finding a practitioner:

- Ask your doctor or other health professionals whether they have recommendations or are willing to make a referral.

- Ask someone you believe to be knowledgeable about CAM if they can recommend a practitioner for the type of therapy you are seeking.

- Contact a nearby hospital or a medical school and ask if they maintain a list of area CAM practitioners or could make a recommendation.

About This Chapter: Information in this chapter is excerpted from "Selecting a Complementary and Alternative Medicine (CAM) Practitioner," National Center for Complementary and Alternative Medicine (NCCAM), National Institutes of Health, NCCAM Publication No. D168, September 2004.

Some regional medical centers may have CAM centers or CAM practitioners on staff.

• Ask if your therapy will be covered by insurance; for example, some insurers cover visits to a chiropractor. If it will, ask for a list of CAM practitioners who accept your insurance.

• Contact a professional organization for the type of practitioner you are seeking. Often, professional organizations have standards of practice, provide referrals to practitioners, have publications explaining the therapy (or therapies) that their members provide, and may offer information on the type of training needed and whether practitioners of a therapy must be licensed or certified in your state. Professional organizations can be located by searching the internet or directories in libraries (ask the librarian). One directory is the Directory of Information Resources On-line (DIRLINE) compiled by the National Library of Medicine (http://dirline.nlm.nih.gov). It contains locations and descriptive information about a variety of health organizations, including CAM associations and organizations. You may find more than one member organization for some CAM professions; this may be because there are different "schools" of practice within the profession or for other reasons.

• Many states have regulatory agencies or licensing boards for certain types of practitioners. They may be able to provide you with information regarding practitioners in your area. Your state, county, or city health department may be able to refer you to such agencies or boards. Licensing, accreditation, and regulatory laws for CAM practices are becoming more common to help ensure that practitioners are competent and provide quality services.

Will insurance cover the cost of a CAM practitioner?

Few CAM therapies are covered by insurance and the amount of coverage offered varies depending upon the insurer. Before agreeing to a treatment that a CAM practitioner suggests, you should check with your insurer to see if they will cover any portion of the therapy's cost. If insurance does cover a portion of the cost, you will want to ask if the practitioner accepts your insurance or participates in your insurer's network. Even with insurance, you may be responsible for a percentage of the cost of therapy.

I have located the names of several practitioners. How do I select one?

Begin by contacting the practitioners on your list and gathering information.

- Ask what training or other qualifications the practitioner has. Ask about her education, additional training, licenses, and certifications. If you contacted a professional organization, see if the practitioner's qualifications meet the standards for training and licensing for that profession.

- Ask if it is possible to have a brief consultation in person or by phone with the practitioner. This will give you a chance to speak with the practitioner directly. The consultation may or may not involve a charge.

- Ask if there are diseases/health conditions in which the practitioner specializes and how frequently he treats patients with problems similar to yours.

- Ask if the practitioner believes the therapy can effectively address your complaint and if there is any scientific research supporting the treatment's use for your condition.

> **✔ Quick Tip**
>
> Before selecting a CAM therapy or practitioner, talk with your primary health care provider(s) or someone you believe to be knowledgeable about CAM. Tell them about the therapy you are considering and ask any questions you may have. They may know about the therapy and be able to advise you on its safety, use, and effectiveness, or possible interactions with medications.

- Ask how many patients the practitioner typically sees in a day and how much time she spends with each patient.

- Ask whether there is a brochure or website to tell you more about the practice.

- Ask about charges and payment options. How much do treatments cost? If you have insurance, does the practitioner accept your insurance or participate in your insurer's network? Even with insurance, you may be responsible for a percentage of the cost.

- Ask about the hours appointments are offered. How long is the wait for an appointment? Consider whether this will be convenient for your schedule.

Remember!!
Communicating with your practitioner(s) can be key to ensuring the best possible health care.

- Ask about office location. If you are concerned, ask about public transportation and parking. If you need a building with an elevator or a wheelchair ramp, ask about them.

- Ask what will be involved in the first visit or assessment.

- Observe how comfortable you feel during these first interactions.

Once you have gathered the information, assess the answers and determine which practitioner was best able to respond to your questions and best suits your needs.

I have selected a practitioner. What questions should I ask at my first visit?

The first visit is very important. Come prepared to answer questions about your health history, such as surgeries, injuries, and major illnesses, as well as prescriptions, vitamins, and other supplements you take. Not only will the practitioner wish to gather information from you, but you will want to ask questions, too. Write down ahead of time the questions you want to ask, or take a family member or friend with you to help you remember the questions and answers. Some people bring a tape recorder to record the appointment. (Ask the practitioner for permission to do this in advance.) Here are some questions you may want to ask:

- What benefits can I expect from this therapy?

- What are the risks associated with this therapy?

- Do the benefits outweigh the risks for my disease or condition?

- What side effects can be expected?

- Will the therapy interfere with any of my daily activities?

- How long will I need to undergo treatment? How often will my progress or plan of treatment be assessed?

- Will I need to buy any equipment or supplies?

- Do you have scientific articles or references about using the treatment for my condition?

- Could the therapy interact with conventional treatments?

- Are there any conditions for which this treatment should not be used?

How do I know if the practitioner I have selected is right for me?

After your first visit with a practitioner, evaluate the visit. Ask yourself these questions:

- Was the practitioner easy to talk to? Did the practitioner make me feel comfortable?

- Was I comfortable asking questions? Did the practitioner appear willing to answer them, and were they answered to my satisfaction?

- Was the practitioner open to how both CAM therapy and conventional medicine might work together for my benefit?

- Did the practitioner get to know me and ask me about my condition?

- Did the practitioner seem knowledgeable about my specific health condition?

- Does the treatment recommended seem reasonable and acceptable to me?

- Was the practitioner clear about the time and costs associated with treatment?

Can I change my mind about the treatment or the practitioner?

Yes, if you are not satisfied or comfortable, you can look for a different practitioner or stop treatment. However, as with any conventional treatment, talk with your practitioner before stopping to make sure that it is safe to simply stop treatment. It may not be advisable to stop some therapies midway through a course of treatment.

Discuss with your practitioner the reasons you are not satisfied or comfortable with treatment. If you decide to stop a therapy or seek another practitioner, make sure that you share this information with any other health care practitioners you may have, as this will help them make decisions about your care.

Part Two

Whole Medical Systems

Chapter 5

Whole Medical Systems: An Overview

Whole medical systems involve complete systems of theory and practice that have evolved independently from or parallel to allopathic (conventional) medicine. Many are traditional systems of medicine that are practiced by individual cultures throughout the world. Major Eastern whole medical systems include traditional Chinese medicine (TCM) and Ayurvedic medicine, one of India's traditional systems of medicine. Major Western whole medical systems include homeopathy and naturopathy. Other systems have been developed by Native American, African, Middle Eastern, Tibetan, and Central and South American cultures.

Traditional Chinese Medicine

TCM is a complete system of healing that dates back to 200 B.C. in written form. Korea, Japan, and Vietnam have all developed their own unique versions of traditional medicine based on practices originating in China. In the TCM view, the body is a delicate balance of two opposing and inseparable forces—yin and yang. Yin represents the cold, slow, or passive principle, while yang represents the hot, excited, or active principle. Among the major assumptions in TCM are that health is achieved by maintaining the body in a "balanced state" and that disease is due to an internal imbalance of

About This Chapter: Information in this chapter is from "Whole Medical Systems: An Overview," National Center for Complementary and Alternative Medicine (NCCAM), National Institutes of Health, NCCAM Publication No. D236, October 2004.

yin and yang. This imbalance leads to blockage in the flow of qi (or vital energy) and of blood along pathways known as meridians. TCM practitioners typically use herbs, acupuncture, and massage to help unblock qi and blood in patients in an attempt to bring the body back into harmony and wellness.

Treatments in TCM are typically tailored to the subtle patterns of disharmony in each patient and are based on an individualized diagnosis. The diagnostic tools differ from those of conventional medicine. There are three main therapeutic modalities:

1. Acupuncture and moxibustion (moxibustion is the application of heat from the burning of the herb moxa at the acupuncture point)

2. *Chinese Materia Medica* (the catalog of natural products used in TCM)

3. Massage and manipulation

Although TCM proposes that natural products cataloged in Chinese Materia Medica or acupuncture can be used alone to treat virtually any illness, quite often they are used together, and sometimes in combination with, other modalities (e.g., massage, moxibustion, diet changes, or exercise).

The scientific evidence on selected modalities from TCM is discussed below.

Acupuncture

The report from a Consensus Development Conference on Acupuncture held at the National Institutes of Health (NIH) in 1997 states that acupuncture is being "widely" practiced by thousands of acupuncturists, physicians, dentists, and other practitioners for relief or prevention of pain and for various other health conditions. In terms of the evidence at that time, acupuncture was considered to have potential clinical value for nausea/vomiting and dental pain, and limited evidence suggested its potential in the treatment of other pain disorders, paralysis and numbness, movement disorders, depression, insomnia, breathlessness, and asthma.

Preclinical studies have documented acupuncture's effects, but they have not been able to fully explain how acupuncture works within the framework of the Western system of medicine.

It is proposed that acupuncture produces its effects by the conduction of electromagnetic signals at a greater-than-normal rate, thus aiding the activity of pain-killing biochemicals, such as endorphins and immune system cells at specific sites in the body. In addition, studies have shown that acupuncture may alter brain chemistry by changing the release of neurotransmitters and neurohormones and affecting the parts of the central nervous system related to sensation and involuntary body functions, such as immune reactions and processes whereby a person's blood pressure, blood flow, and body temperature are regulated.

Chinese Materia Medica

Chinese Materia Medica is a standard reference book of information on medicinal substances that are used in Chinese herbal medicine. Herbs or botanicals usually contain dozens of bioactive compounds. Many factors, such as geographic location, harvest season, post-harvest processing, and storage, could have a significant impact on the concentration of bioactive compounds. In many cases, it is not clear which of these compounds underlie an herb's medical use. Moreover, multiple herbs are usually used in combinations called formulas in TCM, which makes the standardization of herbal preparations very difficult. Further complicating research on TCM herbs, herbal compositions and the quantity of individual herbs in a classic formula are usually adjusted in TCM practice according to individualized diagnoses.

❖ **It's A Fact!!**

In the traditional Chinese medicine view, the body is a delicate balance of two opposing and inseparable forces—yin and yang. Yin represents the cold, slow, or passive principle, while yang represents the hot, excited, or active principle.

In the past decades, major efforts have been made to study the effects and effectiveness of single herbs and of combinations of herbs used in classic TCM formulas. The following are examples of such work:

- *Artemisia annua:* Ancient Chinese physicians identified that this herb controls fevers. In the 1970s, scientists extracted the chemical artemisinin from *Artemisia annua*. Artemisinin is the starting material for the semi-synthetic artemisinins that are proven to treat malaria and are widely used.

- *Tripterygium wilfordii Hook F* (**Chinese Thunder God vine**): Thunder God vine has been used in TCM for the treatment of autoimmune and inflammatory diseases. The first small randomized, placebo-controlled trial of a Thunder God vine extract in the United States showed a significant dose-dependent response in patients with rheumatoid arthritis. In larger, uncontrolled studies, however, renal, cardiac, hematopoietic, and reproductive toxicities of Thunder God vine extracts have been observed.

Ayurvedic Medicine

Ayurveda, which literally means "the science of life," is a natural healing system developed in India. Ayurvedic texts claim that the sages who developed India's original systems of meditation and yoga developed the foundations of this medical system. It is a comprehensive system of medicine that places equal emphasis on the body, mind, and spirit, and strives to restore the innate harmony of the individual. Some of the primary Ayurvedic treatments include diet, exercise, meditation, herbs, massage, exposure to sunlight, and controlled breathing. In India, Ayurvedic treatments have been developed for various diseases (e.g., diabetes, cardiovascular conditions, and neurological disorders). However, a survey of the Indian medical literature indicates that the quality of the published clinical trials generally falls short of contemporary methodological standards with regard to criteria for randomization, sample size, and adequate controls.

Naturopathy

Naturopathy is a system of healing, originating from Europe, that views disease as a manifestation of alterations in the processes by which the body naturally heals itself. It emphasizes health restoration as well as disease treatment. The term "naturopathy" literally translates as "nature disease." Today naturopathy, or naturopathic medicine, is practiced throughout Europe, Australia, New Zealand, Canada, and the United States. There are six principles that form the basis of naturopathic practice in North America (not all are unique to naturopathy):

✤ **It's A Fact!!**

Naturopathy views disease as a manifestation of alterations in the processes by which the body naturally heals itself.

1. The healing power of nature

2. Identification and treatment of the cause of disease

3. The concept of "first do no harm"

4. The doctor as teacher

5. Treatment of the whole person

6. Prevention

The core modalities supporting these principles include diet modification and nutritional supplements, herbal medicine, acupuncture and Chinese medicine, hydrotherapy, massage and joint manipulation, and lifestyle counseling. Treatment protocols combine what the practitioner deems to be the most suitable therapies for the individual patient.

Virtually no research studies on naturopathy as a complete system of medicine have been published. A limited number of studies on botanicals in the context of use as naturopathic treatments have been published. For example, in a study of 524 children, echinacea did not prove effective in treating colds. In contrast, a smaller, double-blind trial of an herbal extract solution containing echinacea, propolis (a resinous product collected from beehives), and vitamin C for ear pain in 171 children concluded that the extract may be beneficial for ear pain associated with acute otitis media. A naturopathic extract known as Otikon Otic Solution (containing *Allium sativum, Verbascum thapsus, Calendula flores,* and *Hypericum perforatum* in olive oil) was found as effective as anesthetic ear drops and was proven appropriate for the management of acute otitis media-associated ear pain. Another study looked at the clinical effectiveness and cost-effectiveness of naturopathic cranberry tablets versus cranberry juice and versus a placebo as prophylaxis against urinary tract infections (UTIs). Compared with the placebo, both cranberry juice and cranberry tablets decreased the number of UTIs. Cranberry tablets proved to be the most cost-effective prevention for UTIs.

Homeopathy

Homeopathy is a complete system of medical theory and practice. Its founder, German physician Samuel Christian Hahnemann (1755–1843), hypothesized that one can select therapies on the basis of how closely symptoms produced by a remedy match the symptoms of the patient's disease. He called this the "principle of similars." Hahnemann proceeded to give repeated doses of many common remedies to healthy volunteers and carefully record the symptoms they produced. This procedure is called a "proving" or, in modern homeopathy, a "human pathogenic trial." As a result of this experience, Hahnemann developed his treatments for sick patients by matching the symptoms produced by a drug to symptoms in sick patients. Hahnemann emphasized from the beginning carefully examining all aspects of a person's health status, including emotional and mental states, and tiny idiosyncratic characteristics.

Since homeopathy is administered in minute or potentially nonexistent material dosages, there is skepticism in the scientific community about its efficacy. Nonetheless, the medical literature provides evidence of ongoing research in the field. Studies of homeopathy's effectiveness involve three areas of research:

1. Comparisons of homeopathic remedies and placebos

2. Studies of homeopathy's effectiveness for particular clinical conditions

3. Studies of the biological effects of potencies, especially ultra-high dilutions

Five systematic reviews and meta-analyses evaluated clinical trials of the effectiveness of homeopathic remedies as compared with placebo. The reviews found that, overall, the quality of clinical research in homeopathy is low. But when high-quality studies were selected for analysis, a surprising number showed positive results.

Overall, clinical trial results are contradictory, and systematic reviews and meta-analyses have not found homeopathy to be a definitively proven treatment for any medical condition.

♣ **It's A Fact!!**
In homeopathy's view, one can select therapies on the basis of how closely symptoms produced by a remedy match the symptoms of the patient's disease.

Summary

While whole medical systems differ in their philosophical approaches to the prevention and treatment of disease, they share a number of common elements. These systems are based on the belief that one's body has the power to heal itself. Healing often involves marshaling multiple techniques that involve the mind, body, and spirit. Treatment is often individualized and dependent on the presenting symptoms. To date, the National Center for Complementary and Alternative Medicine's (NCCAM) research efforts have focused on individual therapies with adequate experimental rationale and not on evaluating whole systems of medicine as they are commonly practiced.

Chapter 6

Ayurvedic Medicine

Ayurvedic medicine (also called Ayurveda) is one of the world's oldest medical systems. It originated in India and has evolved there over thousands of years. In the United States, Ayurveda is considered complementary and alternative medicine (CAM)—more specifically, a CAM whole medical system. Many therapies used in Ayurveda are also used on their own as CAM—for example, herbs, massage, and yoga. This chapter will introduce you to Ayurveda's major ideas and practices.

What is Ayurvedic medicine?

Ayurvedic medicine is also called Ayurveda. It is a system of medicine that originated in India several thousand years ago. The term Ayurveda combines two Sanskrit words—*ayur*, which means life, and *veda*, which means science or knowledge. Ayurveda means "the science of life."

In the United States, Ayurveda is considered a type of CAM and a whole medical system. As with other such systems, it is based on theories of health and illness and on ways to prevent, manage, or treat health problems. Ayurveda aims to integrate and balance the body, mind, and spirit (thus, some view it as "holistic"). This balance is believed to lead to contentment and health, and to help prevent illness. However, Ayurveda also proposes treatments for

About This Chapter: Information in this chapter is from "What is Ayurvedic Medicine," National Center for Complementary and Alternative Medicine (NCCAM), National Institutes of Health, NCCAM Publication No. D287, October 2005.

specific health problems, whether they are physical or mental. A chief aim of Ayurvedic practices is to cleanse the body of substances that can cause disease, and this is believed to help reestablish harmony and balance.

What is the history of Ayurvedic medicine?

Ayurveda is based on ideas from Hinduism, one of the world's oldest and largest religions. Some Ayurvedic ideas also evolved from ancient Persian thoughts about health and healing.

Many Ayurvedic practices were handed down by word of mouth and were used before there were written records. Two ancient books, written in Sanskrit on palm leaves more than 2,000 years ago, are thought to be the first texts on Ayurveda—Caraka Samhita and Susruta Samhita. They cover many topics, which include the following:

- Pathology (the causes of illness)

- Diagnosis

- Treatment

- Surgery (this is no longer part of standard Ayurvedic practice)

- How to care for children

- Lifestyle

- Advice for practitioners, including medical ethics

- Philosophy

> ♣ **It's A Fact!!**
> In Ayurvedic philosophy, people, their health, and the universe are all thought to be related. It is believed that health problems can result when these relationships are out of balance.

Ayurveda has long been the main system of health care in India, although conventional (Western) medicine is becoming more widespread there, especially in urban areas. About 70 percent of India's population lives in rural areas; about two-thirds of rural people still use Ayurveda and medicinal plants to meet their primary health care needs. In addition, most major cities have an Ayurvedic college and hospital. Ayurveda and variations of it have also been practiced for centuries in Pakistan, Nepal, Bangladesh, Sri Lanka, and Tibet. The professional practice of Ayurveda in the United States began to grow and became more visible in the late 20th century.

How common is the use of Ayurveda in the United States?

The first national data to answer this question are from a survey released in May 2004 by the National Center for Health Statistics and the National Center for Complementary and Alternative Medicine (NCCAM). More than 31,000 adult Americans were surveyed about their use of CAM, including specific CAM therapies such as Ayurveda. Among the respondents, four-tenths of 1 percent had ever used Ayurveda, and one-tenth of 1 percent had used it in the past 12 months. When these percentages are adjusted to nationally representative numbers, about 751,000 people in the United States had ever used Ayurveda, and 154,000 people had used it within the past 12 months.

What major beliefs underlie Ayurveda?

Here is a summary of major beliefs in Ayurveda that pertain to health and disease.

Interconnectedness

Ideas about the relationships among people, their health, and the universe form the basis for how Ayurvedic practitioners think about problems that affect health. Ayurveda holds the following beliefs:

- All things in the universe (both living and nonliving) are joined together.

- Every human being contains elements that can be found in the universe.

- All people are born in a state of balance within themselves and in relation to the universe.

- The processes of life disrupt this state of balance. Disruptions can be physical, emotional, spiritual, or a combination. Imbalances weaken the body and make the person susceptible to disease.

- Health will be good if one's interaction with the immediate environment is effective and wholesome.

- Disease arises when a person is out of harmony with the universe.

Constitution And Health

Ayurveda also has some basic beliefs about the body's constitution. "Constitution" refers to a person's general health, how likely he is to become out of balance, and his ability to resist and recover from disease or other health problems. An overview of these beliefs is as follows:

- The constitution is called the prakriti. The prakriti is thought to be a unique combination of physical and psychological characteristics and the way the body functions. It is influenced by such factors as digestion and how the body deals with waste products. The prakriti is believed to be unchanged over a person's lifetime.

- Three qualities called doshas form important characteristics of the constitution, and control the activities of the body. Practitioners of Ayurveda call the doshas by their original Sanskrit names: vata, pitta, and kapha. The following is also believed:

  - Each dosha is made up of one or two of the five basic elements: space, air, fire, water, and earth.

  - Each dosha has a particular relationship to body functions and can be upset for different reasons.

  - A person has her own balance of the three doshas, although one dosha usually is prominent. Doshas are constantly being formed and reformed by food, activity, and bodily processes.

  > **✤ It's A Fact!!**
  >
  > Practitioners expect patients to be active participants in their treatment, because many Ayurvedic treatments require changes in diet, lifestyle, and habits.

  - Each dosha is associated with a certain body type, a certain personality type, and a greater chance of certain types of health problems.

  - An imbalance in a dosha will produce symptoms that are related to that dosha and are different from symptoms of an imbalance in another dosha. An unhealthy lifestyle or diet; too much or too little mental and physical exertion; or not being properly protected from the weather, chemicals, or germs may cause imbalances.

In summary, it is believed that a person's chances of developing certain types of diseases are related to the way doshas are balanced, the state of the physical body, and mental or lifestyle factors.

What is each dosha like?

Here are some important beliefs about the three doshas:

• The vata dosha is thought to be a combination of the elements space and air. It is considered the most powerful dosha because it controls very basic body processes such as cell division, the heart, breathing, and the mind. Vata can be thrown out of balance by, for example, staying up late at night, eating dry fruit, or eating before the previous meal is digested. People with vata as their main dosha are thought to be especially susceptible to skin, neurological, and mental diseases.

• The pitta dosha represents the elements fire and water. Pitta is said to control hormones and the digestive system. When pitta is out of balance, a person may experience negative emotions (such as hostility and jealousy) and have physical symptoms (such as heartburn within 2 or 3 hours of eating). Pitta is upset by, for example, eating spicy or sour food; being angry, tired, or fearful; or spending too much time in the sun. People with a predominantly pitta constitution are thought to be susceptible to heart disease and arthritis.

• The kapha dosha combines the elements water and earth. Kapha is thought to help keep up strength and immunity and to control growth. An imbalance in the kapha dosha may cause nausea immediately after eating. Kapha is aggravated by, for example, sleeping during the daytime, eating too many sweet foods, eating after one is full, and eating and drinking foods and beverages with too much salt and water (especially in the springtime). Those with a predominant kapha dosha are thought to be vulnerable to diabetes, gallbladder problems, stomach ulcers, and respiratory illnesses such as asthma.

How does an Ayurvedic practitioner decide on a person's dosha balance?

Practitioners seek to determine the primary dosha and the balance of doshas through questions that allow them to become very familiar with the patient. Not all questions have to do with particular symptoms. The practitioner will do the following:

- Ask about diet, behavior, lifestyle practices, and the reasons for the most recent illness and symptoms the patient had

- Carefully observe such physical characteristics as teeth, skin, eyes, and weight

- Take a person's pulse, because each dosha is thought to make a particular kind of pulse

How else does an Ayurvedic practitioner work with the patient at first?

In addition to questioning, Ayurvedic practitioners use observation, touch, therapies, and advising. During an examination, the practitioner checks the patient's urine, stool, tongue, bodily sounds, eyes, skin, and overall appearance. He will also consider the person's digestion, diet, personal habits, and resilience (ability to recover quickly from illness or setbacks). As part of the effort to find out what is wrong, the practitioner may prescribe some type of treatment. The treatment is generally intended to restore the balance of one particular dosha. If the patient seems to improve as a result, the practitioner will provide additional treatments intended to help balance that dosha.

How does an Ayurvedic practitioner treat health problems?

The practitioner will develop a treatment plan and may work with people who know the patient well and can help. This helps the patient feel emotionally supported and comforted, which is considered important.

In general, treatments use several approaches, often more than one at a time. These are the goals of treatment:

- **Eliminate impurities.** A process called panchakarma is intended to be cleansing; it focuses on the digestive tract and the respiratory system. For

> ♣ **It's A Fact!!**
> **Treatment Goals**
> - Eliminate impurities
> - Reduce symptoms
> - Reduce worry and increase harmony in the patient's life
> - Help eliminate both physical and psychological problems

the digestive tract, cleansing may be done through enemas, fasting, or special diets. Some patients receive medicated oils through a nasal spray or inhaler. This part of treatment is believed to eliminate worms or other agents thought to cause disease.

• **Reduce symptoms.** The practitioner may suggest various options, including yoga exercises, stretching, breathing exercises, meditation, and lying in the sun. The patient may take herbs (usually several), often with honey, with the intent to improve digestion, reduce fever, and treat diarrhea. Sometimes foods such as lentil beans or special diets are also prescribed. Very small amounts of metal and mineral preparations also may be given, such as gold or iron. Careful control of these materials is intended to protect the patient from harm.

• **Reduce worry and increase harmony in the patient's life.** The patient may be advised to seek nurturing and peacefulness through yoga, meditation, exercise, or other techniques.

• **Help eliminate both physical and psychological problems.** Vital points therapy and/or massage may be used to reduce pain, lessen fatigue, or improve circulation. Ayurveda proposes that there are 107 "vital points" in the body where life energy is stored, and that these points may be massaged to improve health. Other types of Ayurvedic massage use medicinal oils.

How are plant products used in Ayurvedic treatment?

In Ayurveda, the distinction between food and medicine is not as clear as in Western medicine. Food and diet are important components of Ayurvedic practice, and so there is a heavy reliance on treatments based on herbs and plants, oils (such as sesame oil), common spices (such as turmeric), and other naturally occurring substances.

Currently, some 5,000 products are included in the "pharmacy" of Ayurvedic treatments. In recent years, the Indian government has collected and published safety information on a small number of them. Historically, plant compounds have been grouped into categories according to their effects. For example, some compounds are thought to heal, promote vitality, or relieve pain. The compounds are described in many texts prepared through national medical agencies in India.

Below are a few examples of how some botanicals (plants and their products) have been or are currently used in treatment. In some cases, these may be mixed with metals.

- The spice turmeric has been used for various diseases and conditions, including rheumatoid arthritis, Alzheimer's disease, and wound healing.

- A mixture (Arogyawardhini) of sulfur, iron, powdered dried fruits, tree root, and other substances has been used to treat problems of the liver.

- An extract from the resin from a tropical shrub (*Commiphora mukul*, or guggul) has been used for a variety of illnesses. In recent years, there has been research interest in its use to possibly lower cholesterol.

In the United States, how are Ayurvedic practitioners trained and certified?

Practitioners of Ayurveda in the United States have various types of training. Some are trained in the Western medical tradition (such as medical or nursing school) and then study Ayurveda. Others may have training in naturopathic medicine, a whole medical system, either before or after their Ayurvedic training. Many study in India, where there are more than 150 undergraduate and more than 30 postgraduate colleges for Ayurveda. This training can take up to 5 years.

Students who receive all of their Ayurvedic training in India can earn either a bachelor's or doctoral degree. After graduation, they may go to the United States or other countries to practice. Some practitioners are trained in a particular aspect of Ayurvedic practice—for example, massage or meditation—but not in others, such as preparing botanical treatments.

The United States has no national standard for certifying or training Ayurvedic practitioners, although a few states have approved Ayurvedic schools. Some Ayurvedic professional organizations are collaborating to develop licensing requirements.

Consumers interested in Ayurveda should be aware that not every practitioner offering services or treatments called "Ayurvedic" has been trained in an Ayurvedic medical school. Services offered at spas and salons, for example, often fall into this category. If you are seeking Ayurvedic medical treatment, it is important to ask about the practitioner's training and experience.

❧ It's A Fact!!
About Dietary Supplements

Dietary supplements were defined in a law passed by Congress in 1994. A dietary supplement must meet all of the following conditions:

- It is a product (other than tobacco) intended to supplement the diet, which contains one or more of the following: vitamins; minerals; herbs or other botanicals; amino acids; or any combination of the above ingredients.

- It is intended to be taken in tablet, capsule, powder, soft gel, gel cap, or liquid form.

- It is not represented for use as a conventional food or as a sole item of a meal or the diet.

- It is labeled as being a dietary supplement.

Here is some other important information about dietary supplements:

- They are regulated as foods, not drugs, so there could be quality issues in the manufacturing process.

- Supplements can interact with prescribed or over-the-counter medicines and other supplements.

- Natural does not necessarily mean safe or effective.

- Consult your health care provider before starting a supplement, especially if you are pregnant or nursing, or considering giving a supplement to a child.

Does Ayurveda work?

Ayurveda includes many types of therapies and is used for many health issues. However, very few rigorous, controlled scientific studies have been carried out on Ayurvedic practices. In India, the government began systematic research in 1969, and the work continues.

Are there concerns about Ayurvedic medicine?

Health officials in India and other countries have expressed concerns about certain Ayurvedic practices, especially those involving herbs, metals, minerals, or other materials. Here are some of those concerns:

• Ayurvedic medications have the potential to be toxic. Many materials used in them have not been thoroughly studied in either Western or Indian research. In the United States, Ayurvedic medications are regulated as dietary supplements, a category of foods. As such, they are not required to meet the rigorous standards for conventional medicines. An American study published in 2004 found that of 70 Ayurvedic remedies purchased over-the-counter (all had been manufactured in South Asia), 14 (one-fifth) contained lead, mercury, and/or arsenic at levels that could be harmful. Also in 2004, the Centers for Disease Control and Prevention received 12 reports of lead poisoning linked to the use of Ayurvedic medications.

• Most Ayurvedic medications consist of combinations of herbs and other medicines, so it can be challenging to know which ones are having an effect and why.

• Whenever two or more medications are used, there is the potential for them to interact with each other. As a result, the effectiveness of at least one may increase or decrease in the body. For example, it is known that guggul lipid (an extract of guggul) may increase the activity of aspirin, which could lead to bleeding problems.

• Most clinical trials of Ayurvedic approaches have been small, had problems with research designs, lacked appropriate control groups, or had other issues that affected how meaningful the results were.

♣ It's A Fact!!

In Ayurveda, herbs, metals, massage, and other products and techniques are used with the intent of cleansing the body and restoring balance. Some of these products may be harmful when used on their own or when used with conventional medicines.

What should people do if they are considering or using Ayurveda?

• Tell your health care provider if you are considering or using Ayurveda or another CAM therapy. This is for your safety and a comprehensive treatment plan. Women who are pregnant or nursing, or people who are thinking of using CAM to treat a child, should be sure to consult their provider.

• It is important to make sure that any diagnosis of a disease or condition has been made by a provider who has substantial conventional medical training and experience with managing that disease or condition.

• Proven conventional treatments should not be replaced with an unproven CAM treatment.

• It is better to use Ayurvedic remedies under the supervision of an Ayurvedic medicine practitioner than to try to treat yourself.

• Ask about the practitioner's training and experience.

• Tell your provider(s) about any dietary supplements or medications (prescription or over-the-counter) you are using or considering. Prescribed medicines may need to be adjusted if you are also using a CAM therapy. Also, herbal supplements can have safety issues.

• Find out whether any rigorous scientific studies have been done on the therapies you are interested in.

Is NCCAM supporting any studies on Ayurveda?

Yes, NCCAM supports studies in this area. Here are some examples:

• Researchers at the University of Pennsylvania School of Medicine tested the effects of guggul lipid on high cholesterol. Over the 6-month period of this study, they did not find that adults with high cholesterol showed any improvement in cholesterol levels. In fact, the levels of low-density lipoproteins (the "bad" cholesterol) increased slightly in some people in the group taking guggul. In addition, some in the guggul lipid group developed a skin rash. This team is conducting further studies on herbal therapies used in Ayurveda for cardiovascular conditions, including curcuminoids (substances found in the root of the plant turmeric).

• At the NCCAM-supported Center for Phytomedicine Research at the University of Arizona, scientists are investigating three botanicals (ginger, turmeric, and boswellia) used in Ayurvedic medicine to treat inflammatory disorders. They are seeking to better understand these botanicals and determine whether they might be useful in treating arthritis and asthma.

• A compound from a plant called *Mucuna pruriens*, also known as cowhage, is being studied at the Cleveland Clinic Foundation. The research team is investigating the compound's potential to prevent or lessen the severe, often disabling side effects that people with Parkinson's disease experience from prolonged treatment with conventional drugs.

Chapter 7

Homeopathy

Homeopathy ("home-ee-AH-pah-thy"), also known as homeopathic medicine, is a form of health care that developed in Germany and has been practiced in the United States since the early 19th century. Homeopathic practitioners are commonly called homeopaths.

What is homeopathy?

The term homeopathy comes from the Greek words homeo, meaning similar, and pathos, meaning suffering or disease. Homeopathy is an alternative medical system. Alternative medical systems are built upon complete systems of theory and practice, and often have evolved apart from and earlier than the conventional medical approach used in the United States. Homeopathy takes a different approach from conventional medicine in diagnosing, classifying, and treating medical problems.

Key concepts of homeopathy include the following:

- Homeopathy seeks to stimulate the body's defense mechanisms and processes so as to prevent or treat illness.

- Treatment involves giving very small doses of substances called remedies

About This Chapter: Information in this chapter is excerpted from "Questions and Answers About Homeopathy," National Center for Complementary and Alternative Medicine (NCCAM), National Institutes of Health, NCCAM Publication No. D183, April 2003.

that, according to homeopathy, would produce the same or similar symptoms of illness in healthy people if they were given in larger doses.

- Treatment in homeopathy is individualized (tailored to each person). Homeopathic practitioners select remedies according to a total picture of the patient, including not only symptoms, but also lifestyle, emotional and mental states, and other factors.

♣ It's A Fact!!

In homeopathy, a key premise is that every person has energy called a vital force or self-healing response. When this energy is disrupted or imbalanced, health problems develop. Homeopathy aims to stimulate the body's own healing responses.

What is the history of the discovery and use of homeopathy?

In the late 1700s, Samuel Hahnemann, a physician, chemist, and linguist in Germany, proposed a new approach to treating illness. This was at a time when the most common medical treatments were harsh, such as bloodletting, purging, blistering, and the use of sulfur and mercury. At the time, there were few effective medications for treating patients, and knowledge about their effects was limited.

Hahnemann was interested in developing a less threatening approach to medicine. The first major step reportedly was when he was translating an herbal text and read about a treatment (cinchona bark) used to cure malaria. He took some cinchona bark and observed that, as a healthy person, he developed symptoms that were very similar to malaria symptoms. This led Hahnemann to consider that a substance may create symptoms that it can also relieve. This concept is called the "similia principle" or "like cures like." The similia principle had a prior history in medicine, from Hippocrates in Ancient Greece—who noted for example, that recurrent vomiting could be treated with an emetic (such as ipecacuanha) that would be expected to make it worse—to folk medicine. Another way to view "like cures like" is that symptoms are part of the body's attempt to heal itself; for example, a fever can develop as a result of an immune response to an infection, a cough may help to eliminate mucus, and medication may be given to support this self-healing response.

Hahnemann tested single, pure substances on himself and, in more dilute forms, on healthy volunteers. He kept meticulous records of his experiments and participants' responses, and he combined these observations with information from clinical practice, the known uses of herbs and other medicinal substances, and toxicology, eventually treating the sick and developing homeopathic clinical practice.

Hahnemann added two additional elements to homeopathy:

- A concept that became "potentization," which holds that systematically diluting a substance, with vigorous shaking at each step of dilution, makes the remedy more, not less, effective by extracting the vital essence of the substance. If dilution continues to a point where the substance's molecules are gone, homeopathy holds that the "memory" of them—that is, the effects they exerted on the surrounding water molecules—may still be therapeutic.

- A concept that treatment should be selected based upon a total picture of an individual and his symptoms, not solely upon symptoms of a disease. Homeopaths evaluate not only a person's physical symptoms but also her emotions, mental states, lifestyle, nutrition, and other aspects. In homeopathy, different people with the same symptoms may receive different homeopathic remedies.

Hans Burch Gram, a Boston-born doctor, studied homeopathy in Europe and introduced it into the United States in 1825. European immigrants trained in homeopathy also made the treatment increasingly available in America. In 1835, the first homeopathic medical college was established in Allentown, Pennsylvania. By the turn of the 20th century, 8 percent of all American medical practitioners were homeopaths, and there were 20 homeopathic medical colleges and more than 100 homeopathic hospitals in the United States.

In the late 19th and early 20th centuries, numerous medical advances were made, such as the recognition of the mechanisms of disease, Pasteur's germ theory, the development of antiseptic techniques, and the discovery of ether anesthesia. In addition, a report (the so-called "Flexner Report") was released that triggered major changes in American medical education.

Homeopathy was among the disciplines negatively affected by these developments. Most homeopathic medical schools closed down, and by the 1930s others had converted to conventional medical schools.

In the 1960s, homeopathy's popularity began to revive in the United States. According to a 1999 survey of Americans and their health, over 6 million Americans had used homeopathy in the preceding 12 months. The World Health Organization noted in 1994 that homeopathy had been integrated into the national health care systems of numerous countries, including Germany, the United Kingdom, India, Pakistan, Sri Lanka, and Mexico. Several schools of practice exist within homeopathy.

Persons using homeopathy do so to address a range of health concerns, from wellness and prevention to treatment of injuries, diseases, and conditions. Studies have found that many people who seek homeopathic care seek it for help with a chronic medical condition. Many users of homeopathy treat themselves with homeopathic products and do not consult a professional.

What kind of training do homeopathic practitioners receive?

In European countries, training in homeopathy is usually pursued either as a primary professional degree completed over 3 to 6 years or as postgraduate training for doctors.

In the United States, training in homeopathy is offered through diploma programs, certificate programs, short courses, and correspondence courses. Also, homeopathic training is part of medical education in naturopathy. Most homeopathy in the United States is practiced along with another health care practice for which the practitioner is licensed, such as conventional medicine, naturopathy, chiropractic, dentistry, acupuncture, or veterinary medicine (homeopathy is used to treat animals).

> ♣ **It's A Fact!!**
> Homeopathic treatment involves giving extremely small doses of substances that produce characteristic symptoms of illness in healthy people when given in larger doses. This approach is called "like cures like."

Laws about what is required to practice homeopathy vary among states. Three states (Connecticut, Arizona, and Nevada) license medical doctors specifically for homeopathy.

What do homeopathic practitioners do in treating patients?

Typically, in homeopathy, patients have a lengthy first visit, during which the provider takes an in-depth assessment of the patient. This is used to guide the selection of one or more homeopathic remedies. During follow-up visits, patients report how they are responding to the remedy or remedies, which helps the practitioner make decisions about further treatment.

What are homeopathic remedies?

Most homeopathic remedies are derived from natural substances that come from plants, minerals, or animals. A remedy is prepared by diluting the substance in a series of steps, as mentioned previously. Homeopathy asserts that this process can maintain a substance's healing properties regardless of how many times it has been diluted. Many homeopathic remedies are so highly diluted that not one molecule of the original natural substance remains. Remedies are sold in liquid, pellet, and tablet forms.

How does the U.S. Food and Drug Administration (FDA) regulate homeopathic remedies?

Because of their long use in the United States, the U.S. Congress passed a law in 1938 declaring that homeopathic remedies are to be regulated by the FDA in the same manner as nonprescription, over-the-counter (OTC) drugs, which means that they can be purchased without a physician's prescription. Today, although conventional prescription drugs and new OTC drugs must undergo thorough testing and review by the FDA for safety and effectiveness before they can be sold, this requirement does not apply to homeopathic remedies.

Remedies are required to meet certain legal standards for strength, quality, purity, and packaging. In 1988, the FDA required that all homeopathic remedies list the indications for their use (i.e., the medical problems to be treated) on the label. The FDA also requires the label to list ingredients, dilutions, and instructions for safe use.

The guidelines for homeopathic remedies are found in an official guide, the *Homeopathic Pharmacopoeia of the United States*, which is authored by a nongovernmental, nonprofit organization of industry representatives and homeopathic experts. The *Pharmacopoeia* also includes provisions for testing new remedies and verifying their clinical effectiveness. Remedies on the market before 1962 have been accepted into the *Homeopathic Pharmacopoeia of the United States* based on historical use, rather than scientific evidence from clinical trials.

Have any side effects or complications been reported from the use of homeopathy?

The FDA has learned of a few reports of illness associated with the use of homeopathic remedies. However, the FDA reviewed these reports and decided that the remedies were not likely to be the cause, because of the high dilutions.

Here is some general information that has been reported about risks and side effects in homeopathy:

- Homeopathic medicines in high dilutions, taken under the supervision of trained professionals, are considered safe and unlikely to cause severe adverse reactions.

- Some patients report feeling worse for a brief period of time after starting homeopathic remedies. Homeopaths interpret this as the body temporarily stimulating symptoms while it makes an effort to restore health.

- Liquid homeopathic remedies can contain alcohol and are permitted to have higher levels of alcohol than conventional drugs for adults. This may be of concern to some consumers. However, no adverse effects from the alcohol levels have been reported either to the FDA or in the scientific literature.

- Homeopathic remedies are not known to interfere with conventional drugs; however, if you are considering using homeopathic remedies, you should discuss this with your health care provider. If you have more than one provider, discuss it with each one.

As with all medicinal products, a person taking a homeopathic remedy is best advised to do the following:

- Contact his health care provider if his symptoms continue unimproved for more than 5 days.

- Keep the remedy out of the reach of children.

- Consult a health care provider before using the product if the user is a woman who is pregnant or nursing a baby.

What has scientific research found out about whether homeopathy works?

The results of individual, controlled clinical trials of homeopathy have been contradictory. In some trials, homeopathy appeared to be no more helpful than a placebo; in other studies, some benefits were seen that the researchers believed were greater than one would expect from a placebo.

Are there scientific controversies associated with homeopathy?

Yes. Homeopathy is an area of complementary and alternative medicine (CAM) that has seen high levels of controversy and debate, largely because a number of its key concepts do not follow the laws of science (particularly chemistry and physics). These are some of the controversies:

- It is debated how something that causes illness might also cure it.

- It has been questioned whether a remedy with a very tiny amount (perhaps not even one molecule) of active ingredient could have a biological effect, beneficial or otherwise.

- Effects in homeopathy might be due to the placebo or other non-specific effect.

- There are key questions about homeopathy that are yet to be subjected to studies that are well-designed, such as whether it actually works for some of the diseases or medical conditions for which it is used, and if so, how it might work.

- There is a point of view that homeopathy does work, but that modern scientific methods have not yet explained why. The failure of science to provide full explanations for all treatments is not unique to homeopathy.

• Some people feel that if homeopathy appears to be helpful and safe, then scientifically valid explanations or proofs of this alternative system of medicine are not necessary.

Is the National Center for Complementary and Alternative Medicine (NCCAM) funding research on homeopathy?

Yes. NCCAM supports a number of studies in this area. Here are some examples:

• Homeopathy for physical, mental, and emotional symptoms of fibromyalgia (a chronic disorder involving widespread musculoskeletal pain, multiple tender points on the body, and fatigue)

• Homeopathy for brain deterioration and damage in animal models for stroke and dementia

• The homeopathic remedy cadmium, to find out whether it can prevent damage to the cells of the prostate when those cells are exposed to toxins.

✎ What's It Mean?

Bloodletting: A healing practice used for many centuries. In bloodletting, incisions were made in the body to drain a quantity of blood, in the belief that this would help drain out the "bad blood" or sickness.

Naturopathy: Also, known as naturopathic medicine, it is an alternative medical system that emphasizes natural healing approaches (such as herbs, nutrition, and movement or manipulation of the body). Some elements of naturopathy are similar to homeopathy, such as an intent to support the body's own self-healing response.

Placebo: Is designed to resemble as much as possible the treatment being studied in a clinical trial, except that the placebo is inactive. An example of a placebo is a pill containing sugar instead of the drug or other substance being studied.

Toxicology: The science of the effects of chemicals on human health.

Chapter 8

Naturopathic Medicine

What is Naturopathic Medicine?

Founded upon a holistic philosophy, naturopathic medicine combines safe and effective traditional therapies with the most current advances in modern medicine. Naturopathic medicine is appropriate for the management of a broad range of health conditions affecting all people of all ages.

Naturopathic physicians (NDs) are the highest trained practitioners in the broadest scope of naturopathic medical modalities. In addition to the basic medical sciences and conventional diagnostics, naturopathic education includes therapeutic nutrition, botanical medicine, homeopathy, natural childbirth, classical Chinese medicine, hydrotherapy, naturopathic manipulative therapy, pharmacology and minor surgery.

Philosophy

Naturopathic physicians are primary care and specialty doctors who address the underlying cause of disease through effective, individualized natural therapies that integrate the healing powers of body, mind, and spirit.

About This Chapter: "What Is Naturopathic Medicine?" "Philosophy," "History of Naturopathic Medicine," and "Practice Modalities," © American Association of Naturopathic Physicians. Reprinted with permission. Available online at http://www.naturopathic.org, accessed November 2005.

Naturopathic physicians are unique in providing diagnosis and treatment that bridges both conventional and natural medicine perspectives. They integrate scientific research with the healing powers of nature.

The goal of a naturopathic physician is to employ therapies that support and promote the body's natural healing process, leading to the highest state of wellness.

As professional leaders and pioneers in science-based natural medicine, naturopathic physicians advocate the development of professional standards, accountability, and regulation of all forms of medicine in all jurisdictions to maintain public safety and freedom of choice in health care. They support broad inclusion, collaboration, and equal access in the health care system at all levels.

The American Association of Naturopathic Physicians, in Washington, D.C., is the national organization of the profession.

♣ It's A Fact!!
Definition Of A Naturopathic Doctor

Diagnoses, treats, and cares for patients, using system of practice that bases treatment of physiological functions and abnormal conditions on natural laws governing the human body. Utilizes physiological, psychological, and mechanical methods, such as air, water, light, heat, earth, phytotherapy, food and herb therapy, psychotherapy, electrotherapy, physiotherapy, minor and orificial surgery, mechanotherapy, naturopathic corrections and manipulation, and natural methods or modalities, together with natural medicines, natural processed foods, and herbs and nature's remedies. Excludes major surgery, therapeutic use of x-ray and radium, and use of drugs, except those assimilable substances containing elements or compounds which are components of body tissues and are physiologically compatible to body processes for maintenance of life.

Source: From the *Dictionary of Occupational Titles, Revised Fourth Edition*, 1991, United States Department of Labor.

History Of Naturopathic Medicine

Naturopathic medicine, sometimes called "naturopathy," is as old as healing itself and as new as the latest discoveries in biochemical sciences. In the United States, the naturopathic medical profession's infrastructure is based on accredited educational institutions, professional licensing by a growing number of states, national standards of practice and care, peer review, and an ongoing commitment to state-of-the-art scientific research. Modern American naturopathic physicians receive extensive training in and use therapies that are primarily natural (hence the name naturopathic) and nontoxic, including clinical nutrition, homeopathy, botanical medicine, hydrotherapy, physical medicine, and counseling. Many NDs have additional training and certification in acupuncture and home birthing. These contemporary NDs, who have attended naturopathic medical colleges recognized by the U.S. Department of Education, practice medicine as primary health care providers and are increasingly acknowledged as leaders in bringing about progressive changes in the nation's medical system.

The word "naturopathy" was first used in the U.S. exactly 100 years ago. But the natural therapies and the philosophy on which naturopathy is based have been effectively used to treat diseases since ancient times. As Rene Dubos noted in *The Mirage of Health* (1959), the word "physician" is from the Greek root meaning "nature." Hippocrates, a physician who lived 2,400 years ago, is often considered the earliest predecessor of naturopathic physicians, particularly in terms of his teaching that "nature is healer of all diseases" and his formulation of the concept *vis medicatrix naturae*—"the healing power of nature." This concept has long been at the core of indigenous medicine in many cultures around the world and remains one of the central themes of naturopathic philosophy to this day.

The earliest doctors and healers worked with herbs, foods, water, fasting, and tissue manipulation—gentle treatments that do not obscure the body's own healing powers. Today's naturopathic physicians continue to use these therapies as their main tools and to advocate a healthy dose of primary prevention. In addition, modern NDs conduct and make practical use of the latest biochemical research involving nutrition, botanicals, homeopathy, and other natural treatments.

For many diseases and conditions (a few examples are ulcerative colitis, asthma, menopause, flu, obesity, and chronic fatigue), treatments used by naturopathic physicians can be primary and even curative. Naturopathic physicians also function within an integrated framework, for example referring patients to an appropriate medical specialist such as an oncologist or a surgeon. Naturopathic therapies can be employed within that context to complement the treatments used by conventionally trained medical doctors. The result is a team-care approach that recognizes the needs of the patient to receive the best overall treatment most appropriate to his or her specific medical condition.

Recent History

Naturopathic medicine was popular and widely available throughout the U.S. well into the early part of the 20th century. Around 1920, from coast to coast, there were a number of naturopathic medical schools, thousands of naturopathic physicians, and scores of thousands of patients using naturopathic therapies. The rise of "scientific medicine," the discovery and increasing use of "miracle drugs" like antibiotics, the institutionalization of a large medical system primarily based (both clinically and economically) on high-tech and pharmaceutical treatments were all associated by mid-century with the temporary decline of naturopathic medicine and most other methods of natural healing.

By the 1970s, however, the American public was becoming increasingly disenchanted with conventional medicine. The profound clinical limitations of conventional medicine and its out-of-control costs were becoming obvious, and millions of Americans were inspired to look for new options and alternatives. Naturopathy and all of complementary alternative medicine began to enter a new era of rejuvenation.

Looking To The Future

Today, licensed naturopathic physicians are experiencing noteworthy clinical successes, providing leadership in innovative natural medical research, enjoying increasing political influence, and looking forward to an unlimited future potential. Both the American public and policy makers are recognizing and contributing to the resurgence of the comprehensive system of health care practiced by NDs. In 1992, the National Institute of Health's (NIH) Office of Alternative Medicine, created by an act of Congress, invited leading naturopathic physicians (educators, researchers, and clinical practitioners) to serve on key federal advisory panels and to help define priorities and design protocols for state-of-the-art alternative medical research. In 1994, the NIH selected Bastyr University as the national center for research on alternative treatments for HIV/AIDS. At a one-million-dollar level of funding, this action represented the formal recognition by the federal government of the legitimacy and significance of naturopathic medicine.

Meanwhile, the number of new NDs is steadily increasing, and licensure of naturopathic physicians is expanding into new states. By April of 1996, eleven of fifty states had naturopathic licensing laws (Alaska, Arizona, Connecticut, Hawaii, Maine, Montana, New Hampshire, Oregon, Utah, Vermont, and Washington). A number of other states are likely to enact naturopathic licensing in the near future.

In October 1996, in a major development for both public health and naturopathic medicine, the Natural Medicine Clinic opened in Kent, Washington. Funded by the King County (Seattle) Department of Public Health, the clinic is the first medical facility in the nation to offer natural medical treatments to people in the community, paid for by tax dollars. Bastyr University, a naturopathic college, was selected over several leading Seattle-area hospitals to operate the clinic.

Practice Modalities

Naturopathic Medicine—Primary Care

Naturopathic physicians (NDs or NMDs) are general practitioners trained as specialists in natural medicine. In practice, naturopathic physicians perform physical examinations, laboratory testing, gynecological exams, nutritional and dietary assessments, metabolic analysis, and allergy testing. They may order x-ray, ultrasounds, other imaging procedures, and other diagnostic tests. They are the only primary care physicians clinically trained in the use of the following wide variety of natural therapeutics.

Clinical Nutrition

Naturopathic physicians understand that what you eat is the basis for your health. Adopting a healthy diet is often the first step towards correcting health problems. Many medical conditions can be treated more effectively with foods and nutritional supplements than they can by other means, but with fewer complications and side effects. Naturopathic physicians may use specific individual diets, fasting, and nutritional supplements with their patients.

> ♣ **It's A Fact!!**
>
> Naturopathic physicians combine and tailor treatments to the needs of the individual in a way that acknowledges the patient as a participant.
>
> Source: "Practice Modalities" © American Association of Naturopathic Physicians.

Botanical Medicine

Plants have powerful healing properties. Many pharmaceutical drugs have their origins in plant substances. Naturopathic physicians use plant substances for their healing effects and nutritional value.

Homeopathic Medicine

This gentle, yet effective system of medicine, is more than 200 years old and is based on the principle that "like cures like." Homeopathic medicines are very small doses of natural substances that can stimulate the body's self-healing response without side effects. Some conditions for which conventional medicine has no effective treatments will respond well to homeopathy.

Physical Medicine

Naturopathic medicine includes methods of therapeutic manipulation for muscles and bones. Naturopathic physicians also employ therapeutic exercise, massage, hydrotherapy, gentle electrical therapies, ultrasound, and heat and cold.

Oriental Medicine

Naturopathic physicians are trained in the fundamentals of Oriental medicine and diagnosis. They use acupuncture, acupressure, and Chinese herbal medicine to promote healing.

Lifestyle Counseling And Stress Management

Mental attitudes and emotional states can be important elements in healing and disease. Naturopathic physicians are trained in counseling, nutritional balancing, stress management, hypnotherapy, and biofeedback. They also attend to environmental and lifestyle factors that affect their patients' health.

Natural Childbirth

Naturopathic physicians, with additional specialty training, provide natural childbirth care in an out-of-hospital setting. They offer prenatal and postnatal care using appropriate diagnostic techniques.

Minor Surgery

As primary care physicians, naturopathic physicians perform in-office minor surgery including repair of superficial wounds and removal of foreign bodies, warts, and cysts with local anesthesia.

Chapter 9

Osteopathic Medicine

Osteopathic medicine is a distinctive form of medical practice in the United States. Osteopathic medicine provides all of the benefits of modern medicine including prescription drugs, surgery, and the use of technology to diagnose disease and evaluate injury. It also offers the added benefit of hands-on diagnosis and treatment through a system of therapy known as osteopathic manipulative medicine. Osteopathic medicine emphasizes helping each person achieve a high level of wellness by focusing on health education, injury prevention, and disease prevention.

Osteopathic medicine was founded in the late 1800s in Kirksville, Missouri by Andrew Taylor Still, M.D., who felt that the medical practices of the day often caused more harm than good. After losing members of his immediate family to meningitis, Still focused on developing a system of medical care that would promote the body's innate ability to heal itself. He called his system of medicine osteopathy, now known as osteopathic medicine.

Osteopathic physicians, also known as D.O.s, work in partnership with their patients. They consider the impact that lifestyle and community have on the health of each individual, and they work to erase barriers to good health. D.O.s are licensed to practice the full scope of medicine in all 50

About This Chapter: Information in this chapter is from "Osteopathic Medicine." © American Association of Colleges of Osteopathic Medicine. Reprinted with permission. Available online at www.aacom.org/om.html, accessed December 10, 2005.

states. They practice in all types of environments including the military, and in all types of specialties from family medicine to obstetrics, surgery, and aerospace medicine.

D.O.s are trained to look at the whole person from their first days of medical school, which means they see each person as more than just a collection of body parts that may become injured or diseased. This holistic approach to patient care means that osteopathic medical students learn how to integrate the patient into the health care process as a partner. They are trained to communicate with people from diverse backgrounds, and they get the opportunity to practice these skills in the classroom with simulated patients.

Because of this whole-person approach to medicine, approximately 60 percent of all D.O.s choose to practice in the primary care disciplines of family practice, general internal medicine, and pediatrics. Approximately 40 percent of all D.O.s go on to specialize in a wide range of practice areas. If the medical specialty exists, you will find D.O.s there.

♣ It's A Fact!!

Approximately 60 percent of all D.O.s choose to practice in the primary care disciplines of family practice, general internal medicine, and pediatrics.

While America's 47,000 D.O.s account for only 5 percent of the country's physicians, they handle approximately 10 percent of all primary care visits. D.O.s also have a strong history of serving rural and underserved areas, often providing their unique brand of compassionate, patient-centered care to some of the most economically disadvantaged members of society.

In addition to studying all of the typical subjects you would expect student physicians to master, osteopathic medical students take approximately 200 additional hours of training in the art of osteopathic manipulative medicine. This system of hands-on techniques helps alleviate pain, restores motion, supports the body's natural functions, and influence the body's structure to help it function more efficiently.

One key concept osteopathic medical students learn is that structure influences function. Thus, if there is a problem in one part of the body's structure, function in that area, and possibly in other areas, may be affected. For example, restriction of motion in the lower ribs, lumbar spine, and abdomen can cause stomach pain with symptoms that mimic irritable bowel syndrome. By using osteopathic manipulative medicine techniques, D.O.s can help restore motion to these areas of the body thus improving gastrointestinal function, oftentimes restoring it to normal.

Another integral tenet of osteopathic medicine is the body's innate ability to heal itself. Many of osteopathic medicine's manipulative techniques are aimed at reducing or eliminating the impediments to proper structure and function so the self-healing mechanism can assume its role in restoring the person to health.

In addition to a strong history of providing high quality patient care, D.O.s conduct clinical and basic science research to help advance the frontiers of medicine and to demonstrate the effectiveness of the osteopathic approach to patient care. Currently, several organizations are involved in osteopathic clinical research in coordination with the national osteopathic research center. The facility's staff develops, facilitates, and conducts multicenter collaborative clinical research studies.

Chapter 10

Traditional Chinese Medicine

Traditional Chinese medicine (TCM) is a system of health care based on the late-twentieth-century standardization of medical practices that originated in China some 2,500 years ago. Two classic medical texts, the *Nei Jing* (compiled from 100 B.C. to 100 A.D.) and the *Nan Jing* (written circa 100 to 200 A.D.) were important early documents that presented the core concepts of TCM, and they have informed generations of scholars and practitioners ever since. These core concepts suggest that disease is the result of imbalances in the flow of the body's vital energy, or qi (pronounced "chee"), and that the human body is a microcosm of the basic natural forces at work in the universe.

As TCM evolved over the centuries, it came to include treatment of disease using acupuncture, herbal medicine, dietary principles, physical manipulation of the body tissues, therapeutic exercise and movement (tai chi), and the mind-body practice of qigong. TCM reached its apex during the Ming dynasty (1368–1644) then gradually declined to the status of a folk practice until 1949. It was then that the government of the People's Republic of China began to exploit the remaining TCM practitioners as a means of making health care accessible to a suffering and underserved population.

While TCM was fading in China it was nevertheless migrating to the rest of the globe as traders, missionaries, and diplomats visited East Asia in the 17th and 18th centuries and returned home with reports and texts of the classical practices. Chinese immigrating to the United States in the 19th century brought other components of traditional practice with them.

It wasn't until 1971, however, that U.S. citizens really became aware of TCM—and of acupuncture in particular. This came about because James Reston, a *New York Times* reporter became stricken with appendicitis while doing a story on a ping-pong tournament in Beijing, and was treated for post-surgical pain with acupuncture. In a front-page *Times* story he wrote, "I've seen the past, and it works!" This exposure came at a time when many Americans were looking for a more holistic, naturalistic approach to health care, and caused quite a stir among the Western medical community. Since then, acupuncture has become a widely accepted form of treatment in the U.S., and other aspects of TCM are gaining supporters as well.

How Traditional Chinese Medicine Works

A typical TCM evaluation will include three components.

The first assesses the balance between yin and yang—complementary but opposing qualities that represent the natural dualities of the world, such as male/female, day/night, and hot/cold.

The second considers the correspondence of the ailment to the five Chinese elements—wood, fire, earth, metal, and water. It is believed that each internal organ and body system is related to an elemental quality and that the body reflects the natural world in this way.

The third determines which organ or metabolic system requires the most support from therapy. Because of this ancient symbolic method of describing the body in natural terms, a TCM diagnosis

♣ **It's A Fact!!**

Practitioners of TCM seek to promote or restore health by diagnosing and treating "disharmonies" or imbalances in the qi, or natural vital energy of the body.

© 2006 WholeHealth Chicago.

✎ What's It Mean?

Acupuncture: A family of procedures involving stimulation of anatomical points on the body by a variety of techniques. The acupuncture technique that has been most studied scientifically involves penetrating the skin with thin, solid, metallic needles that are manipulated by the hands or by electrical stimulation.

Chiropractic: Focuses on the relationship between bodily structure (primarily that of the spine) and function, and how that relationship affects the preservation and restoration of health. Chiropractors use manipulative therapy as an integral treatment tool.

Homeopathy: A belief that "like cures like," meaning that small, highly diluted quantities of medicinal substances are given to cure symptoms, when the same substances given at higher or more concentrated doses would actually cause those symptoms.

Naturopathic: Proposes that there is a healing power in the body that establishes, maintains, and restores health. Practitioners work with the patient with a goal of supporting this power, through treatments such as nutrition and lifestyle counseling, dietary supplements, medicinal plants, exercise, homeopathy, and treatments from traditional Chinese medicine.

Osteopathic: A form of conventional medicine that, in part, emphasizes diseases arising in the musculoskeletal system. There is an underlying belief that all of the body's systems work together, and disturbances in one system may affect function elsewhere in the body. Some osteopathic physicians practice osteopathic manipulation, a full-body system of hands-on techniques to alleviate pain, restore function, and promote health and well-being.

Qigong: A component of traditional Chinese medicine that combines movement, meditation, and regulation of breathing to enhance the flow of qi (an ancient term given to what is believed to be vital energy) in the body, improve blood circulation, and enhance immune function.

Source: "What is Complementary and Alternative Medicine," National Center for Complementary and Alternative Medicine (NCCAM), National Institutes of Health, NCCAM Publication No. D156, May 2002.

can sound like a weather report. Colds and flus may be described as "wind-heat invading the lungs," or "wind-cold affecting the stomach." Some kinds of endometriosis could be described as "damp-heat" in the "lower burner." An asthma patient might have "a failure of the kidneys to moisten the lungs." These descriptive diagnoses can lead some conventional physicians to conclude that TCM is "unscientific," whereas the actual practice of TCM is a sophisticated system based on the practical science of observing and altering the natural functions of the body.

Practitioners of TCM use tools such as acupuncture, massage, qigong, and herbal medicine to restore balance and health to the body. A change in diet may also be recommended. For example, if someone's condition is showing too much dampness and cold, the practitioner may suggest cutting out cold foods such as salads, and recommend drying and warming herbs for dietary support. If the condition is more a physical problem, such as an injury, the treatment may focus on the muscles, nerves, tendons, and circulation at the site of the injury, with acupuncture, massage, and anti-inflammatory herbs all being prescribed.

Chinese herbs are available in the U.S. in liquid, tablet, or powder form and can be prescribed by practitioners familiar with the proper diagnosis of a particular condition. In China, some TCM practitioners specialize in herbal medicines and are expert at modifying and individualizing the classical herbal formulas. These practitioners can artfully construct a mixture from raw herbs or powders to treat disharmonies of the organs as well as any current symptoms.

♣ It's A Fact!!

Chinese herbs are prescribed in most TCM practices. These remedies are often sophisticated and complex mixtures that were developed for organ imbalances and disease support and standardized centuries ago. Those most often used today have been carefully formulated to have minimal side effects.

© 2006 WholeHealth Chicago.

If you plan to take Chinese herbs, make sure any mixtures you use have standardized content and are processed under the direction of a licensed health professional familiar with their medicinal effects. Individualized herbal mixtures should be prescribed only under the advice of a TCM practitioner who has training in herbal drug compounding. A TCM herbal mixture could be as safe as an over-the-counter cold and flu drug mixture, or as powerful as a strong prescription drug.

What You Can Expect

A TCM examination is thorough, but noninvasive. The practitioner will take a careful medical history, noting your body's reaction to stress and your tendencies toward illness symptoms. He will observe the color and form of your face and body, note the condition of your skin and nails, check how your breath and body odor smells, and look at your posture and demeanor. The condition of your tongue—its shape, color, and coating—also provides important data on the way your circulation and metabolism is affecting your internal organs. Your pulse will be felt at three different points on each wrist, each location corresponding to a different part of the body. Considered together, this information gives the practitioner a sense of your body's current functioning.

From this examination, the practitioner will consider the patterns of imbalance in your body and will choose the proper type of treatment for you. Depending on the training of the practitioner, treatment may consist of acupuncture, massage, change in diet, herbal remedies, qigong, or any combination of these.

Duration and frequency of treatment depends on the ailment and the person being treated. Acute problems may require one to three visits over two weeks, whereas a course of acupuncture for a chronic problem may require 12 treatments in three months to see positive results. Herbal tonics for restoring healthy internal organ function may require weeks of use, whereas herbs for colds and flu can show good results in hours. Practitioners with other skills in addition to their TCM training, such as chiropractic, homeopathy, Western physical medicine, and drug therapy, may integrate these treatments with the TCM program.

Health Benefits

The various techniques used in TCM can address a wide range of illnesses. Acupuncture has been shown to be particularly effective in relieving chronic pain, caused by such ailments as arthritis, sinusitis, headache, PMS, and back pain, and has aided postoperative pain as well. It can also ease nausea and other discomforts associated with cancer treatment. In addition, acupuncture has been beneficial in rehabilitation for certain neurologic problems such as stroke. It is also used in treating addiction to cigarettes, alcohol, and other drugs.

Chinese herbal remedies are often used to treat acute ailments such as the flu and the common cold, and are also recommended for chronic conditions such as fibromyalgia, migraine headaches, and irritable bowel syndrome.

Chinese massage techniques, such as anmo and tuina, utilize the same points as acupuncture to unblock qi and ease the stress and tension that often accompanies illness. Anmo involves pressing and rubbing motions; tuina is a thrusting and rolling type of massage.

Many research studies of the various types of TCM are currently ongoing. A 1999 study published in *Clinical and Experimental Obstetrics and Gynecology* showed that acupuncture eased pain following breast cancer surgery. Another recent study in *Alternative Therapies in Health and Medicine* found that practicing tai chi helped improve mobility for people with multiple sclerosis.

A 1998 study published in the *Journal of the American Medical Association* showed that Chinese herbal medicine helped improve the symptoms of irritable bowel syndrome. A group of 116 patients were divided into groups: One group was given an individualized Chinese herbal treatment, one group was given a standard Chinese herbal formulation, and the third group was given a placebo, or dummy pill. The two groups who received the herbs experienced significant improvement in their symptoms (the individualized group maintained the improvement longer), as compared to the placebo group.

Preliminary studies have also been conducted on Chinese herbal treatments and skin conditions. A study published in *Lancet* found that 31 patients with atopic dermatitis appeared to be helped by Chinese herbal therapy.

A review of clinical trials in the *British Journal of Clinical Pharmacology* found two trials that showed Chinese herbs as a more effective treatment than a placebo for treating eczema. More study is needed in this area, however, because some adverse reactions have been reported to the treatment.

How To Choose A Practitioner

In the United States, practitioners typically specialize in a particular component of TCM, such as acupuncture, herbs, or massage, rather than the entire discipline. The regulation of TCM varies from state to state. Acupuncturists are licensed in many states and Doctors of Oriental Medicine (O.M.D.) are licensed in some states to prescribe herbal remedies as well as acupuncture treatments. Many biomedically trained doctors, naturopaths, osteopaths, and chiropractors have studied acupuncture and other branches of TCM and incorporated them into their practices.

Mastering the full range of Chinese medicine is a complex process that requires many years of study and practice. However, medical personnel with less training may still be able to perform acupuncture and herbal medicine safely, by working according to protocols designed by TCM practitioners. As you would with any health provider, check into your TCM practitioner's training and background.

Cautions

If you have a chronic condition or a new acute problem that is seriously disabling you, get a diagnostic evaluation from a conventional primary care physician before consulting an acupuncturist.

Plan on coordinating your care between your biomedical doctor and your acupuncturist. If they won't work together, find ones that will.

Be sure your acupuncturist uses sterile, disposable needles.

As with any health practitioner, if the condition is not improving in a reasonable time, get a second opinion. There are increasing numbers of practitioners familiar with both Western and traditional Chinese medicine, should you need a re-evaluation.

Acupuncturists in California and Nevada must take an exam in order to dispense Chinese herbs. In other states, herbal certification is voluntary. Ask if your acupuncturist has passed the National Certification Commission for Acupuncture and Oriental Medicine herbal exam.

Herbal remedies are regulated as "foodstuffs" under current federal laws. This means that the Food and Drug Administration (FDA) has not evaluated their effectiveness and safety as therapies. Be sure to work only with a licensed and certified practitioner to ensure that you get the best care.

Visit http://www.wholehealthchicago.com for more information.

Reprinted from http://www.WholeHealthChicago.com.

Chapter 11

Traditional Native American Medicine

In Harmony

Perhaps more than any other aspect of American Indian life, Indian cultural beliefs and traditional Indian medicine arouse the nation's curiosity. Derided as pagan witchcraft by European settlers 200 years ago, co-opted by pop culture into "new age" movement today, and dismissed by scientists as nonsense, traditional American Indian health practices are universally misunderstood and oversimplified.

While beliefs, ceremonies, and rituals differ from tribe to tribe around the country, many American Indians share an underlying belief that the natural or correct state of all things is harmony. The beliefs, traditions, and customs handed down through many generations also play a principal role in individual and collective Indian identity. Native Americans strive for a close integration within the family, clan, and tribe, and to live in harmony with their environment. This occurs simultaneously on physical, mental, and spiritual levels; thus, wellness is a state of harmony and balance between mind, body, spirit, and the environment.

About This Chapter: Information under the heading "In Harmony" is excerpted from "Heritage & Health," Indian Health Service, U.S. Department of Health and Human Services, 2005. Text under the heading "Integrating Traditional Native American Medicine With Modern Medicine" is from "When Worlds Collide" by Dana Humphrey, *The New Physician*, November 1997. Reprinted with permission from the American Medical Student Association.

✤ **It's A Fact!!**

The practice of traditional Native American medicine rests on the assumption that sickness and disease represent being out of balance with the natural order of living. Hence the approach to healing is holistic and employs certain ceremonies and rites utilizing herbs and roots to assist the sick in returning to wellness and wholeness.

The patient's family is also asked to be a part of the healing process because achieving wellness most often requires changing one's lifestyle from a negative to a positive way of living. As was the case historically, the traditional healers, the medicine men of today, are highly esteemed in the community, not only in regard to their role and function as healers of the body and mind, but also as community leaders among the people who seek counsel and direction.

Source: Excerpted from "The People," Aberdeen Area, Indian Health Service, U.S. Department of Health and Human Services, November 2004.

Medical treatment provided to a person within this belief system requires integration of their beliefs with modern medical practice. Finding the solution is often a delicate balancing act. The following story illustrates that fine line.

Integrating Traditional Native American Medicine With Modern Medicine

A few years ago, a doctor was called to the hospital bedside of an Apache girl meticulously clad in buckskin. The 11 year-old had developed pneumonia while preparing for what was to be the biggest moment of her young life—the Sunrise Dance. Apache tradition dictates that when a girl has her first menstrual cycle, she is to have an intense, four-day ceremony in which the whole community participates. The timing could not have been worse. In septic shock and on the verge of death, the girl needed to be moved to a city for emergency care; but her grandmother, who oversees preparations for the ritual, stood firm behind her conviction that to miss this rite of passage was the same as death for the girl. The doctor was brought in to negotiate with the tribal chairman. With extended family and hundreds of community members watching, the doctor and the tribal leader decided that the dance would take place on grounds halfway between the hospital and the airstrip where an air transport would be waiting on the runway with engines running. The girl could go ahead with the dance, but the minute she passed out, she was to be flown to Phoenix. The grandmother agreed to the compromise.

On an unusually warm September morning, the ambulance darted into a circle of about 1,000 people at the dance grounds, and the girl was rolled out on a stretcher. "I thought to myself, 'She'll last four minutes,'" the doctor said. Amazingly, the girl stayed conscious and was able to finish the first half of her dance. After a rest stop at the hospital, where she was given penicillin by the doctor and prayed over by her grandmother, she returned to the dance grounds in the afternoon. Once again, with IV and catheter dangling, the girl danced for a while and then went back to the hospital to rest before the evening portion of the ceremony—the most spectacular and important part. That night, with a bonfire blazing and hundreds of people participating in ritual dress, the girl got up, pulled out her IVs and danced for two hours. She spent the night at the hospital and walked out the next morning feeling absolutely fine. "What was it? Our penicillin? The ceremony?" the doctor asked. "I see the grandmother every once in a while, and she just smiles..."

The preceding section is from "When Worlds Collide" by Dana Humphrey, *The New Physician*, November 1997. Reprinted with permission from the American Medical Student Association.

Part Three

Manipulative And Body-Based Practices

Chapter 12

Manipulative And Body-Based Practices: An Overview

Introduction

Under the umbrella of manipulative and body-based practices is a heterogeneous group of CAM interventions and therapies. These include chiropractic manipulation, massage therapy, reflexology, Rolfing, Alexander technique, and a host of others. Surveys of the U.S. population suggest that between 3 percent and 16 percent of adults receive chiropractic manipulation in a given year, while between 2 percent and 14 percent receive some form of massage therapy. In 1997, U.S. adults made an estimated 192 million visits to chiropractors and 114 million visits to massage therapists. Visits to chiropractors and massage therapists combined represented 50 percent of all visits to CAM practitioners. Data on the remaining manipulative and body-based practices are sparser, but it can be estimated that they are collectively used by less than 7 percent of the adult population.

Manipulative and body-based practices focus primarily on the structures and systems of the body, including the bones and joints, the soft tissues, and the circulatory and lymphatic systems. Some practices were derived from

About This Chapter: Information in this chapter is excerpted from "Manipulative and Body-Based Practices: An Overview," National Center for Complementary and Alternative Medicine (NCCAM), National Institutes of Health, NCCAM Publication No. D238, October 2004.

traditional systems of medicine, such as those from China, India, or Egypt, while others were developed within the last 150 years (e.g., chiropractic manipulation). Although many providers have formal training in the anatomy and physiology of humans, there is considerable variation in the training and the approaches of these providers both across and within modalities. For example, chiropractic practitioners, who use primarily manipulations that involve rapid movements, may have a very different treatment approach than massage therapists, whose techniques involve slower applications of force, or than craniosacral therapists. Despite this heterogeneity, manipulative and body-based practices share some common characteristics such as the principles that the human body is self-regulating and has the ability to heal itself and that the parts of the human body are interdependent. Practitioners in all these therapies also tend to tailor their treatments to the specific needs of each patient.

✎ **What's It Mean?**

Alexander technique: Patient education/guidance in ways to improve posture and movement and to use muscles efficiently.

Chiropractic manipulation: Adjustments of the joints of the spine, as well as other joints and muscles.

Craniosacral therapy: Form of massage using gentle pressure on the plates of the patient's skull.

Massage therapy: Assortment of techniques involving manipulation of the soft tissues of the body through pressure and movement.

Osteopathic manipulation: Manipulation of the joints combined with physical therapy and instruction in proper posture.

Reflexology: Method of foot (and sometimes hand) massage in which pressure is applied to "reflex" zones mapped out on the feet (or hands).

Rolfing: Deep tissue massage (also called structural integration).

Research

Primary Challenges Of Research

The primary challenges that have impeded research on the underlying biology of manual therapies include the following:

- Lack of appropriate animal models

- Lack of cross-disciplinary collaborations

- Lack of research tradition and infrastructure at schools that teach manual therapies

- Inadequate use of state-of-the-art scientific technologies

Clinical trials of CAM manual therapies face the same general challenges as trials of procedure-based interventions such as surgery, psychotherapy, or more conventional physical manipulative techniques (e.g., physical therapy). These include the following:

- Identifying an appropriate, reproducible intervention, including dose and frequency. This may be more difficult than in standard drug trials, given the variability in practice patterns and training of practitioners.

- Identifying an appropriate control group(s). In this regard, the development of valid sham manipulation techniques has proven difficult.

- Randomizing subjects to treatment groups in an unbiased manner. Randomization may prove more difficult than in a drug trial, because manual therapies are already available to the public; thus, it is more likely that participants will have a preexisting preference for a given therapy.

- Maintaining investigator and subject compliance to the protocol. Group contamination (which occurs when patients in a clinical study seek additional treatments outside the study, usually without telling the investigators; this will affect the accuracy of the study results) may be more problematic than in standard drug trials, because subjects have easy access to manual therapy providers.

- Reducing bias by blinding subjects and investigators to group assignment. Blinding of subjects and investigators may prove difficult or impossible for certain types of manual therapies. However, the person collecting the outcome data should always be blinded.

- Identifying and employing appropriate validated, standardized outcome measures.

- Employing appropriate analyses, including the intent-to-treat paradigm.

Clinical Studies: Trials

Forty-three clinical trials have been conducted on the use of spinal manipulation for low-back pain, and there are numerous systematic reviews and meta-analyses of the efficacy of spinal manipulation for both acute and chronic low-back pain. These trials employed a variety of manipulative techniques. Overall, manipulation studies of varying quality show minimal to moderate evidence of short-term relief of back pain. Information on cost-effectiveness, dosing, and long-term benefit is scant. Although clinical trials have found no evidence that spinal manipulation is an effective treatment for asthma, hypertension, or dysmenorrhea, spinal manipulation may be as effective as some medications for both migraine and tension headaches and may offer short-term benefits to those suffering from neck pain. Studies have not compared the relative effectiveness of different manipulative techniques.

Although there have been numerous published reports of clinical trials evaluating the effects of various types of massage for a variety of medical conditions (most with positive results), these trials were almost all small, poorly designed, inadequately controlled, or lacking adequate statistical analyses. For example, many trials included co-interventions that made it impossible to evaluate the specific effects of massage, while others evaluated massage delivered by individuals who were not fully trained massage therapists or followed treatment protocols that did not reflect common (or adequate) massage practice.

There have been very few well-designed controlled clinical trials evaluating the effectiveness of massage for any condition, and only three randomized controlled trials have specifically evaluated massage for the condition most frequently treated with massage—back pain. All three trials found massage to be effective, but two of these trials were very small. More evidence is needed.

Risks

There are some risks associated with manipulation of the spine, but most reported side effects have been mild and of short duration. Although rare, incidents of stroke and vertebral artery dissection have been reported following manipulation of the cervical spine. Despite the fact that some forms of massage involve substantial force, massage is generally considered to have few adverse effects. Contraindications for massage include deep vein thrombosis, burns, skin infections, eczema, open wounds, bone fractures, and advanced osteoporosis.

❧ It's A Fact!!

In the United States, manipulative therapy is practiced primarily by doctors of chiropractic, some osteopathic physicians, and physical therapists. Doctors of chiropractic perform more than 90 percent of the spinal manipulations in the United States, and the vast majority of the studies that have examined the cost and utilization of spinal manipulation have focused on chiropractic.

Utilization/Integration

Individual provider experience, traditional use, or arbitrary payer capitation decisions—rather than the results of controlled clinical trials—determine many patient care decisions involving spinal manipulation. More than 75 percent of private payers and 50 percent of managed care organizations provide at least some reimbursement for chiropractic care. Congress has mandated that the Department of Defense (DOD) and the Department of Veterans Affairs provide chiropractic services to their beneficiaries, and there are DOD medical clinics offering manipulative services by osteopathic physicians and physical therapists. The State of Washington has mandated coverage of CAM services for medical conditions normally covered by insurance. The integration of manipulative services into health care has reached this level despite a dearth of evidence about long-term effects, appropriate dosing, and cost-effectiveness.

Although the numbers of Americans using chiropractic and massage are similar, massage therapists are licensed in fewer than 40 states, and massage is much less likely than chiropractic to be covered by health insurance. Like spinal manipulation, massage is most commonly used for musculoskeletal problems. However, a significant fraction of patients seek massage care for relaxation and stress relief.

Cost

A number of observational studies have looked at the costs associated with chiropractic spinal manipulation in comparison with the costs of conventional medical care, with conflicting results. Overall health care expenditures were lower for patients who received chiropractic treatment than for those who received medical care in a fee-for-service environment. Chiropractic spinal manipulation was found to be more expensive than primary medical care, but less expensive than specialty medical care. Two randomized trials comparing the costs of chiropractic care with the costs of physical therapy failed to find evidence of cost savings through chiropractic treatment. The only study of massage that measured costs found that the costs for subsequent back care following massage were 40 percent lower than those following acupuncture or self care, but these differences were not statistically significant.

Patient Satisfaction

Although there are no studies of patient satisfaction with manipulation in general, numerous investigators have looked at patient satisfaction with chiropractic care. Patients report very high levels of satisfaction with chiropractic care. Satisfaction with massage treatment has also been found to be very high.

Chapter 13

Acupressure

Acupressure is a type of bodywork that involves pressing specific points on the body with the fingers, knuckles, and palms (and sometimes the elbows and feet) to relieve pain, reduce stress, and promote general good health. Developed in China some 5,000 years ago, perhaps out of the natural human instinct to hold or rub a place on the body that hurts, acupressure is part of the holistic system of traditional Chinese medicine (TCM) that also includes acupuncture. (Interestingly, the use of acupressure predates acupuncture by some 2,500 years.)

In the United States, acupressure is primarily used to relieve pain, reduce stress, and improve overall well-being. In China, the technique is used more like first-aid. The Chinese typically practice it on themselves or on family members to treat everyday ailments such as colds, headaches, sore muscles, and hangovers. Specialists are consulted for more complicated problems.

While many people prefer to go to a trained therapist to get acupressure treatments, the techniques, once learned, can be performed on oneself or by a friend.

About This Chapter: Information in this chapter is from "Acupressure." © 2006 WholeHealth Chicago. All rights reserved. Reprinted with permission.

How Acupressure Works

Traditional Chinese medicine views health as the constantly changing flow of vital energy, or qi (pronounced "chee") throughout the body. If that flow is hindered, sickness may develop. The goal of acupressure (and acupuncture) is to release blocked energy by stimulating specific points, called acupoints, along the body's 14 primary meridians, or energy channels. Pressing firmly and steadily on the proper acupoints, it is suggested, can promote energy flow to a part of the body that is experiencing disease or discomfort, enabling it to heal itself more readily. While acupuncture involves stimulation with needles, acupressure typically uses only the practitioner's hands to restore the balance of qi.

Although Western science has found no evidence that meridians actually exist in the body, studies do suggest that pressing on acupoints can release endorphins, the body's natural painkillers.

What You Can Expect

During a treatment, which can last anywhere from 15 minutes to nearly an hour depending on the severity of the problem, an acupressure therapist may have you sit or lie on a massage table. Some acupressure therapists will work through clothing; others will ask you to undress (you will be covered with a towel).

The therapist will then locate and work on the specific acupoints that relate to your condition. Pressing a point behind your knee, for example, can help address low back pain. Or pressing a point on the top of the foot may help ease the pain of migraine.

Typically, the therapist will press each point for about three to ten seconds (longer in some cases). The points may be pressed and released repeatedly. If the problem doesn't respond after about 20 to 30 minutes of treatment, acupressure may not be effective for you on that particular day, or for that particular ailment.

After a treatment, you will probably feel looser and more relaxed. You may experience a slight achiness, but you shouldn't be in pain. Within three to eight visits, you should know whether the treatment is working for your ailment. Stress management usually requires a series of about six regular (weekly or monthly) treatments.

There are many different types of acupressure, and each practitioner may draw from a variety of methods. One of the most popular is shiatsu, a Japanese technique based on ancient Chinese principles. Practitioners of Zen shiatsu use their whole bodies as leverage to apply strong pressure. Barefoot shiatsu practitioners bring the feet into play, as well as the hands, to rub and press acupressure points. In the Chinese acupressure variation known as tuina, practitioners use their hands for massage-like kneading motions. Reflexology is a type of acupressure that involves pressure points on the feet and sometimes the hands.

Even if you prefer to do acupressure on yourself, you may wish to see an acupressure practitioner for a visit or two first, particularly if you are addressing a chronic or complex medical problem. These visits can help you learn where the particular acupoints are on your body.

Health Benefit

Many people have reported success using acupressure to relieve pain, reduce muscle tension, and promote relaxation. A number have found the therapy especially helpful for easing back pain and for certain types of headaches, including migraine. Post-operative pain and nausea has been found to

---

✔ Quick Tip

- Never press on an open wound, swollen or inflamed skin, a bruise, surgery scar, varicose vein, or broken bone.

- Avoid acupressure if you have a contagious disease, an infectious skin disease, or a serious heart, kidney, or lung disorder.

- Avoid acupressure in the area of a known tumor.

- Acupressure should not be applied directly over the lymph nodes.

- Certain acupressure points must be avoided during pregnancy.

respond to pressure point massage. Chronic sinusitis sufferers have also found it useful for easing congestion. Although research results are mixed, acupressure is also commonly used for morning sickness, motion sickness, and other types of nausea.

Some people find that treatments improve their overall vitality and well-being.

How To Choose A Practitioner

There is no licensing procedure for acupressure therapists. Because acupressure involves massage, it is important to find someone you feel comfortable with. A word-of-mouth recommendation from a friend or co-worker may be the best place to start. Having a short phone conversation with the therapist before you go in for a visit may help you find out if you at least like the person.

Reprinted from http://www.WholeHealthChicago.com.

Chapter 14

Acupuncture

What is acupuncture?

Acupuncture is one of the oldest, most commonly used medical procedures in the world. Originating in China more than 2,000 years ago, acupuncture began to become better known in the United States in 1971, when *New York Times* reporter James Reston wrote about how doctors in China used needles to ease his pain after surgery.

The term acupuncture describes a family of procedures involving stimulation of anatomical points on the body by a variety of techniques. American practices of acupuncture incorporate medical traditions from China, Japan, Korea, and other countries. The acupuncture technique that has been most studied scientifically involves penetrating the skin with thin, solid, metallic needles that are manipulated by the hands or by electrical stimulation.

How widely is acupuncture used in the United States?

In the past two decades, acupuncture has grown in popularity in the United States. The report from a Consensus Development Conference on Acupuncture held at the National Institutes of Health (NIH) in 1997 stated that acupuncture is being "widely" practiced by thousands of physicians, dentists,

About This Chapter: Information in this chapter is from "Acupuncture," National Center for Complementary and Alternative Medicine (NCCAM), National Institutes of Health, NCCAM Publication No. D003, December 2004.

acupuncturists, and other practitioners for relief or prevention of pain and for various other health conditions. According to the 2002 National Health Interview Survey, the largest and most comprehensive survey of complementary and alternative medicine (CAM) use by American adults to date, an estimated 8.2 million U.S. adults had ever used acupuncture, and an estimated 2.1 million U.S. adults had used acupuncture in the previous year.

What does acupuncture feel like?

Acupuncture needles are metallic, solid, and hair-thin. People experience acupuncture differently, but most feel no or minimal pain as the needles are inserted. Some people are energized by treatment, while others feel relaxed. Improper needle placement, movement of the patient, or a defect in the needle can cause soreness and pain during treatment. This is why it is important to seek treatment from a qualified acupuncture practitioner.

Is acupuncture safe?

The U.S. Food and Drug Administration (FDA) approved acupuncture needles for use by licensed practitioners in 1996. The FDA requires that sterile, nontoxic needles be used and that they be labeled for single use by qualified practitioners only.

Relatively few complications from the use of acupuncture have been reported to the FDA in light of the millions of people treated each year and the number of acupuncture needles used. Still, complications have resulted from inadequate sterilization of needles and from improper delivery of treatments. Practitioners should use a new set of disposable needles taken from a sealed package for each patient and should swab treatment sites with alcohol or another disinfectant before inserting needles. When not delivered properly, acupuncture can cause serious adverse effects, including infections and punctured organs.

Does acupuncture work?

According to the NIH Consensus Statement on Acupuncture, there have been many studies on acupuncture's potential usefulness, but results have been mixed because of complexities with study design and size, as well as difficulties with choosing and using placebos or sham acupuncture. However,

✎ What's It Mean?

Fibromyalgia: A complex chronic condition having multiple symptoms, including muscle pain, fatigue, and tenderness in precise, localized areas, particularly in the neck, spine, shoulders, and hips. People with this syndrome may also experience sleep disturbances, morning stiffness, irritable bowel syndrome, anxiety, and other symptoms.

Meridian: A traditional Chinese medicine term for each of the 20 pathways throughout the body for the flow of qi, or vital energy, accessed through acupuncture points.

Placebo: An inactive pill or sham procedure given to a participant in a research study as part of a test of the effects of another substance or treatment. Scientists use placebos to get a true picture of how the substance or treatment under investigation affects participants.

Preclinical study: A study done to obtain information about a treatment's safety and side effects when given at different doses to animals or to cells grown in the laboratory.

Qi: A Chinese term for vital energy or life force. In traditional Chinese medicine, qi (pronounced "chee") is believed to regulate a person's spiritual, emotional, mental, and physical balance, and to be influenced by the opposing forces of yin and yang.

Traditional Chinese medicine (TCM): A whole medical system that was documented in China by the 3rd century B.C. TCM is based on a concept of vital energy, or qi, that is believed to flow throughout the body. It is proposed to regulate a person's spiritual, emotional, mental, and physical balance and to be influenced by the opposing forces of yin (negative energy) and yang (positive energy). Disease is proposed to result from the flow of qi being disrupted and yin and yang becoming unbalanced. Among the components of TCM are herbal and nutritional therapy, restorative physical exercises, meditation, acupuncture, and remedial massage.

promising results have emerged, showing efficacy of acupuncture, for example, in adult postoperative and chemotherapy nausea and vomiting and in postoperative dental pain. There are other situations, such as addiction, stroke rehabilitation, headache, menstrual cramps, tennis elbow, fibromyalgia, myofascial pain, osteoarthritis, low-back pain, carpal tunnel syndrome, and asthma, in which acupuncture may be useful as an adjunct treatment or an acceptable alternative or be included in a comprehensive management program. An NCCAM-funded study recently showed that acupuncture provides pain relief, improves function for people with osteoarthritis of the knee, and serves as an effective complement to standard care. Further research is likely to uncover additional areas where acupuncture interventions will be useful.

How might acupuncture work?

Acupuncture is one of the key components of the system of traditional Chinese medicine (TCM). In the TCM system of medicine, the body is seen as a delicate balance of two opposing and inseparable forces: yin and yang. Yin represents the cold, slow, or passive principle, while yang represents the hot, excited, or active principle. Among the major assumptions in TCM are that health is achieved by maintaining the body in a "balanced state" and that disease is due to an internal imbalance of yin and yang. This imbalance leads to blockage in the flow of qi (vital energy) along pathways known as meridians. It is believed that there are 12 main meridians and 8 secondary meridians and

✔ **Quick Tip**

Check a practitioner's credentials. An acupuncture practitioner who is licensed and credentialed may provide better care than one who is not. About 40 states have established training standards for acupuncture certification, but states have varied requirements for obtaining a license to practice acupuncture. Although proper credentials do not ensure competency, they do indicate that the practitioner has met certain standards to treat patients through the use of acupuncture.

Do not rely on a diagnosis of disease by an acupuncture practitioner who does not have substantial conventional medical training. If you have received a diagnosis from a doctor, you may wish to ask your doctor whether acupuncture might help.

that there are more than 2,000 acupuncture points on the human body that connect with them.

Preclinical studies have documented acupuncture's effects, but they have not been able to fully explain how acupuncture works within the framework of the Western system of medicine that is commonly practiced in the United States. It is proposed that acupuncture produces its effects through regulating the nervous system, thus aiding the activity of pain-killing biochemicals such as endorphins and immune system cells at specific sites in the body. In addition, studies have shown that acupuncture may alter brain chemistry by changing the release of neurotransmitters and neurohormones and, thus, affecting the parts of the central nervous system related to sensation and involuntary body functions, such as immune reactions and processes that regulate a person's blood pressure, blood flow, and body temperature.

How do I find a licensed acupuncture practitioner?

Health care practitioners can be a resource for referral to acupuncturists. More medical doctors, including neurologists, anesthesiologists, and specialists in physical medicine, are becoming trained in acupuncture, TCM, and other CAM therapies. In addition, national acupuncture organizations (which can be found through libraries or internet search engines) may provide referrals to acupuncturists.

How much will acupuncture cost?

A practitioner should inform you about the estimated number of treatments needed and how much each will cost. If this information is not provided, ask for it. Treatment may take place over a few days or for several weeks or more. Physician acupuncturists may charge more than non-physician practitioners.

Will it be covered by my insurance?

Acupuncture is one of the CAM therapies that are more commonly covered by insurance. However, you should check with your insurer before you start treatment to see whether acupuncture will be covered for your condition and, if so, to what extent. Some insurance plans require preauthorization for acupuncture.

What should I expect during my first visit?

During your first office visit, the practitioner may ask you at length about your health condition, lifestyle, and behavior. The practitioner will want to obtain a complete picture of your treatment needs and behaviors that may contribute to your condition. Inform the acupuncturist about all treatments or medications you are taking and all medical conditions you have.

Chapter 15

Alexander Technique

The Alexander technique is a method of movement and alignment that teaches people to use their bodies more efficiently. It helps individuals improve their posture, let go of muscle tension, and move with greater ease.

The originator of this technique was Frederick Matthias Alexander (1869–1955), an Australian actor who suffered bouts of hoarseness on stage. When medications and rest failed to help him, Alexander found his career in jeopardy. Using mirrors, he observed that the way he lowered his head and tensed his neck muscles when he recited his lines was restricting his vocal cords. He realized these habits were so ingrained that they had probably become second nature to him. He worked hard to correct his posture, and found that when he did so, his voice was restored. Based on this personal success, Alexander created his eponymous technique around 1896 and published his first book about it, *Man's Supreme Inheritance*, around 1910.

Alexander was so successful that other actors and artists, George Bernard Shaw among them, sought his help. Eventually he stopped acting and created a formal program to promote his method. Today the Alexander technique is taught all over the world. Many performing arts schools incorporate Alexander's precepts into their curricula, and athletes also use it to help prevent injury. In addition, people suffering from back problems and other types of chronic pain have turned to Alexander's methods to ease their discomfort and to improve postural habits.

How The Alexander Technique Works

The philosophy behind the Alexander technique is that the correct relationship between the head, neck, and spine is critical to good health. Proponents of the technique call this three-way relationship "primary control" because they believe it is key to maintaining proper posture, breath, and movement.

♣ **It's A Fact!!**

The goal of this technique is to eradicate such poor habits as slouching and tensing (which can lead to pain, decreased mobility, and other health problems) and replace them with good postural habits.

An incorrect position of the head in relation to the neck and spine, for example, can create muscle tension and cause pain. Once a person's head, neck, and spine are brought into proper alignment, however, the rest of the body should "fall into place." Not only can muscle tension and pain be reduced, according to Alexander practitioners, but some bodily functions, such as breathing and movement, may become easier and more natural as well.

What You Can Expect

You can learn the Alexander technique privately or as part of a group. At a lesson, which lasts about 45 minutes, the instructor will observe the way you walk, stand, sit, lay, and bend. (You should wear loose clothing so you won't feel restricted.) You will be coached to relax your neck muscles so your head balances freely on top of your neck and allows your back to lengthen.

Through verbal instruction and gentle touch, the instructor will then teach you to improve your posture during a variety of everyday activities, such as sitting at a desk and talking on the phone. A poor habit, such as cradling the phone between your head and shoulder (which can put your neck out of alignment) will be replaced with a good habit, such as sitting upright with your shoulders straight while holding the phone to your ear.

Instructors, who are encouraged to be nonjudgmental and supportive, typically recommend one-on-one tutoring to tailor the Alexander technique more fully to your personal activities. If you are a dancer, for example, the instructor may work with you on improving your dance movements; if you are a tennis player, the teacher may coach you on maintaining proper form while you play.

The instructors then encourage you to apply what you have learned to events in your daily life. Gradually, sometimes with as few as six to eight lessons, students can begin to use their bodies more effectively.

Health Benefits

Better body awareness and posture, improved coordination, decreased tension, and more efficient movement have all been credited to the Alexander technique. In addition, for many, it improves overall physical and mental health.

People suffering from chronic neck and back pain, and other painful conditions such as arthritis and fibromyalgia, report finding relief after learning the Alexander technique. Also, the technique may help stress-related problems such as migraines and anxiety attacks.

It is important to note that there have been very few science-based studies evaluating the Alexander technique, and therapeutic claims are primarily anecdotal.

How To Choose A Practitioner

Look for an instructor who is certified by the North American Society of Teachers of the Alexander Technique. To earn this certification, instructors must complete at least three years of training in the technique. Alexander Technique International in Cambridge, Massachusetts, can refer you to a certified instructor.

Cautions

When taught by a qualified instructor, the Alexander technique is safe for everyone, even pregnant women. In fact, many pregnant women report that the technique helps them adjust to the changes their bodies are going through and relieve some of the pressure their growing bellies are putting on their spines.

Reprinted from http://www.WholeHealthChicago.com.

Chapter 16

Applied Kinesiology

What is applied kinesiology?

Applied kinesiology (AK) is a form of diagnosis using muscle testing as a primary feedback mechanism to examine how a person's body is functioning. When properly applied, the outcome of an AK diagnosis will determine the best form of therapy for the patient. Since AK draws together the core elements of many complementary therapies, it provides an interdisciplinary approach to health care.

In general, the applied kinesiologist finds a muscle that tests weak and then attempts to determine why that muscle is not functioning properly. The practitioner will then evaluate and apply the therapy that will best eliminate the muscle weakness and help the patient.

Therapies utilized can include specific joint manipulation or mobilization, various myofascial therapies, cranial techniques, meridian therapy, clinical nutrition, dietary management and various reflex procedures.

In some cases, the examiner may test for environmental or food sensitivities by using a previously strong muscle to find what weakens it.

About This Chapter: Information in this chapter is from "What Is Applied Kinesiology," and "Applied Kinesiology Logo," accessed November 7, 2005 © International College of Applied Kinesiology-USA. Reprinted with permission. For additional information, contact ICAK-USA at 6405 Metcalf Ave., Suite 503, Shawnee Mission, Kansas 66202-3929, (913) 384-5336, or visit their website at http://www.icakusa.com.

Applied kinesiology uses the triad of health—chemical, mental, and structural factors—to describe the proper balance of the major health categories.

The triad is represented by an equilateral triangle with structural health as its base and the upright sides representing chemical and mental health. When a person experiences poor health, it is due to an imbalance in one or more of these three factors.

The triad of health is interactive and all sides must be evaluated for the underlying cause of a problem. A health problem on one side of the triad can affect the other sides. For example, a chemical imbalance may cause mental symptoms. Applied kinesiology enables the practitioner to evaluate the triad's balance and direct therapy toward the imbalanced side or sides.

What is the International College of Applied Kinesiology (ICAK)?

The origin of applied kinesiology is traced to 1964 when George J. Goodheart, Jr., D.C., first observed that postural distortion (for example head tilt, high shoulder, high hip) is usually associated with muscles that test weak. He found that by applying the appropriate therapy, the muscle would test strong and the postural distortion would change.

The College was founded in 1976 by a group of doctors who had been teaching others in applied kinesiology. The purpose of the College is to promote

---

♣ It's A Fact!!
A Brief History Of Applied Kinesiology

During the 1960s, a new system of evaluation began to develop in chiropractic. Dr. George Goodheart of Detroit, Michigan, found that evaluation of normal and abnormal body function could be accomplished by using muscle tests. Since the original discovery, the principle has broadened to include evaluation of the nervous, vascular, and lymphatic systems, nutrition, acupuncture, and cerebrospinal fluid function. This system is called "applied kinesiology" (kih-nee'-see-awl'-oh-jee) or AK.

Source: "A Brief History of Applied Kinesiology," accessed November 7, 2005 © International College of Applied Kinesiology-USA. Reprinted with permission. For additional information, contact ICAK-USA at 6405 Metcalf Ave., Suite 503 Shawnee Mission, Kansas 66202-3929, (913) 384-5336, or visit their website at http://www.icakusa.com.

research and the teaching of AK. It is a professional association dedicated to bringing together doctors and students with common interests and goals.

What is the educational background of an applied kinesiologist?

It takes hundreds of hours of study and years of practice to perfect the multitude of diagnostic techniques that have been developed in AK. In fact, any AK practitioner will tell you that she/he is constantly refining and developing manual muscle testing skills and the interpretation of the test results.

At first glance, muscle testing appears easy, fascinating, and impressive. The ability to test muscles, however, requires specific techniques, sensitivity, and objectivity. Once the muscle testing skill has been developed, it becomes necessary to interpret the outcome of the test. Interpreting the results requires the years of training that qualifies one as a licensed physician. Therefore, applied kinesiology is only taught to persons licensed to diagnose in the health care field.

To practice AK, one must take a basic course that takes over 100 hours of classroom study and practice to complete. A basic proficiency exam in AK must be passed at the end of the course. A minimum of 300 hours of AK instruction, passage of written and oral examinations, and submission of two original research papers are required to reach the next step—becoming a diplomate of the International Board of Applied Kinesiology (DIBAK). A diplomate represents the highest level of certification in AK.

Does applied kinesiology replace standard examinations?

Applied kinesiology is used in addition to standard diagnostics to help determine the cause of a health problem. For example, with certain conditions like hypoglycemia, there will be muscle patterns of weakness or strength found with AK. However, these same patterns could be present because of another nervous system problem such as disease or some type of adaptation.

Only an adequate history of the person, together with standard examination procedures and laboratory findings, will indicate the proper treatment course. Therefore, people performing a simple muscle test and diagnosing what vitamins are needed or other information about health without standard examination is inappropriate. This is making health decisions well beyond what a simple muscle test can determine and actually may be harmful.

The determination of your need for dietary supplements requires knowledge of your symptoms along with an examination for known physical signs of imbalances and a dietary history. Blood, urine, saliva, or stool analyses may be added to the foregoing. An applied kinesiology examination provides additional information and can help to determine what is missing and needs supplementation. Using applied kinesiology, a doctor can often determine which of the many available laboratory tests are the most appropriate to be performed. This can result in a more effective diagnosis while at the same time reducing health care costs.

What is meant by structure?

An important part of applied kinesiology examination is postural analysis. Postural distortion is body language revealing dysfunction. The characteristics of poor posture lead the examiner to various deficiencies in health. Postural analysis is much more than just observing the carriage of the body. It reveals to the examiner improper nerve control that may result in many types of health problems.

Applied kinesiology is a receptor based examination of the nervous and other systems that control or influence health. Postural distortions are often the cause of nerve improper receptor stimulation throughout the body. Postural analysis may reveal an unlevel head on the neck. This inappropriately stimulates nerve receptors controlling muscle organization of body function. The shoulders, arms, trunk, pelvis, and legs are considered in the analysis. Is one shoulder higher or more forward than the other? Is one arm rotated internally more that the other? Is the pelvis level? Finally the feet and their function are evaluated. Like the head on neck reflexes, feet have nerve receptors that may be improperly stimulated causing health problems almost anywhere in the body. An applied kinesiologist may find the cause of a person's shoulder pain, headache or back pain coming from foot dysfunction. As corrections are obtained the posture improves, removing strain that may be causing improper nerve receptor stimulation.

What is the triad of health?

The equilateral triad of health (structure, chemical, mental) is not unique to applied kinesiology. The discoverer of chiropractic, D.D. Palmer, and many others described the triad. The triad represents aspects that influence health, which can be lost or gained through any side of the triad. Physicians of all types tend to concentrate their efforts on only one side of the triad, based primarily on their initial education. Because of the interplay between the sides of the triad, an examination cannot be considered adequate unless all sides of the triad are considered.

Structure

The base of the triad is structure, re-emphasizing its importance in AK. Direct trauma is often what brings a patient to a doctor specializing in structure. Doctors specializing in structure are usually orthopedists and chiropractors. If the problem is acute trauma, such as a lifting injury causing a sacroiliac subluxation or disc herniation, correction by manipulation or surgery often successfully concludes treatment of the case. Chronic postural distortion is body language providing the applied kinesiologist information during the examination.

What appears to be a structural problem may originate from another side of the triad. An example is a sacroiliac subluxation occurring or recurring because of poor support from a weak sartorius muscle due to adrenal gland dysfunction. The sartorius muscle supports the pelvis, and when weak, allows the structural distortion to occur. This muscle is associated with the adrenal gland in the applied kinesiology muscle-organ/gland association. Examining all sides of the triad by applied kinesiology methods finds these interactions.

Chemical

The allopathic physician dominates the chemical side of the triad. Nutritionists are rapidly developing more presence in this area. The difference between the two is that the allopath uses chemicals and other substances to control the body, while the nutritionist uses natural dosages to provide the raw material the body needs to build healthy tissue or maintain health. When the nutritionist uses mega dosages of nutrition, it is similar to using nutrition as medicine, as in the allopathic approach.

Often the chemically oriented physician tries to control the other sides of the triad by medications, such as muscle relaxants and analgesics for structural faults or antidepressants for the mental side. Neither addresses the cause of the problem.

Mental

Psychiatrists, psychologists, and counselors of various types have dominated the mental side of the triad. Chiropractors and other physicians who have a strong "personality dominated" practice often influence this side of the triad.

Many conditions treated by drugs respond to the balanced approach of applied kinesiology. One example is attention deficit disorder (ADD). It is much better to return the nervous system to normal than influence it by drugs.

Interplay Within The Triad

The longer a condition is present, the more likely there will be more than one side of the triad affected. Applied kinesiologists often smile to themselves as a patient relates being treated with an antidepressant for an unrelenting chronic health problem. This often happens when "all tests were normal" and the physician observes the patient's obvious depression about the long-term problem. Sure, the patient is depressed after months or years of the continuing problem. Who wouldn't be? But the depression is not the cause of the problem. The depression is the condition moving into another side of the triad of health. In all conditions, all three sides of the triad should be considered for interplay between them.

Chapter 17

Chiropractic Medicine

What is chiropractic?

The word "chiropractic" combines the Greek words *cheir* (hand) and *praxis* (action) and means "done by hand." Chiropractic is an alternative medical system and takes a different approach from conventional medicine in diagnosing, classifying, and treating medical problems.

The basic concepts of chiropractic can be described as follows:

• The body has a powerful self-healing ability.

• The body's structure (primarily that of the spine) and its function are closely related, and this relationship affects health.

• Chiropractic therapy is given with the goals of normalizing this relationship between structure and function and assisting the body as it heals.

What is the history of the discovery and use of chiropractic?

Chiropractic is a form of spinal manipulation, which is one of the oldest healing practices. Spinal manipulation was described by Hippocrates in ancient Greece. In 1895, Daniel David Palmer founded the modern profession

About This Chapter: Information in this chapter is excerpted from "About Chiropractic and Its Use in Treating Low-Back Pain," National Center for Complementary and Alternative Medicine (NCCAM), National Institutes of Health, NCCAM Publication No. D196, November 2003.

of chiropractic in Davenport, Iowa. Palmer was a self-taught healer and a student of healing philosophies of the day. He observed that the body has a natural healing ability that he believed was controlled by the nervous system. He also believed that subluxations, or misalignments of the spine, interrupt or interfere with this "nerve flow." Palmer suggested that if an organ does not receive its normal supply of impulses from the nerves, it could become diseased. This line of thinking led him to develop a procedure to "adjust" the vertebrae, the bones of the spinal column, with the goal of correcting subluxations.

Some chiropractors continue to view subluxation as central to chiropractic health care. However, other chiropractors no longer view the subluxation theory as a unifying theme in health and illness or as a basis for their practice. Other theories as to how chiropractic might work have been developed.

Who uses chiropractic and for what health problems?

In 1997, it was estimated that Americans made nearly 192 million visits a year to chiropractors. Over 88 million of those visits were to treat back or neck pain. In one recent survey, more than 40 percent of patients receiving chiropractic care were being treated for back or low-back problems. More than half of those surveyed said that their symptoms were chronic. Conditions commonly treated by chiropractors include back pain, neck pain, headaches, sports injuries, and repetitive strains. Patients also seek treatment of pain associated with other conditions, such as arthritis.

Low-back pain is a common medical problem, occurring in up to one-quarter of the population each year. Most people experience significant back pain at least once during their lifetime. Several recent reviews on low-back pain have noted that in most cases acute low-back pain gets better in several weeks, no matter what treatment is used. Often, the cause of back pain is unknown, and it varies greatly in terms of how people experience it and how professionals diagnose it. This makes back pain challenging to study.

What kinds of training do chiropractors receive?

Chiropractic training is a 4-year academic program consisting of both classroom and clinical instruction. At least 3 years of preparatory college work are required for admission to chiropractic schools. Students who graduate receive the degree of Doctor of Chiropractic (D.C.) and are eligible to take state licensure board examinations in order to practice. Some schools also offer postgraduate courses, including 2- to 3-year residency programs in specialized fields.

The Council on Chiropractic Education, an agency certified by the U.S. Department of Education, is the accrediting body for chiropractic colleges in the United States.

What do chiropractors do in treating patients?

If you become a chiropractic patient, during your initial visit the chiropractor will take your health history. He will perform a physical examination, with special emphasis on the spine, and possibly other examinations or tests such as x-rays. If he determines that you are an appropriate candidate for chiropractic therapy, he will develop a treatment plan.

When the chiropractor treats you, he may perform one or more adjustments. An adjustment (also called a manipulation treatment) is a manual therapy, or therapy delivered by the hands. Given mainly to the spine, chiropractic adjustments involve applying a controlled, sudden force to a joint. They are done to increase the range and quality of motion in the area being treated. Other health care professionals, including physical therapists, sports medicine doctors, orthopedists, physical medicine specialists, doctors of osteopathic medicine, doctors of naturopathic medicine, and massage therapists, perform various types of manipulation. In the United States, chiropractors perform over 90 percent of manipulative treatments.

Most chiropractors use other treatments in addition to adjustment, such as mobilization, massage, and non-manual treatments.

Have side effects or problems been reported from using chiropractic to treat back pain?

Patients may or may not experience side effects from chiropractic treatment. Effects may include temporary discomfort in parts of the body that were treated, headache, or tiredness. These effects tend to be minor and to resolve within 1 to 2 days.

The rate of serious complications from chiropractic has been debated. There have been no organized prospective studies on the number of serious complications. From what is now known, the risk appears to be very low. It appears to be higher for cervical-spine, or neck, manipulation (e.g., cases of stroke have been reported). The rare complication of concern from low-back adjustment is cauda equina syndrome, estimated to occur once per millions of treatments (the number of millions varies; one study placed it at 100 million).

For your safety, it is important to inform all of your health care providers about any care or treatments that you are using or considering, including chiropractic. This is to help ensure a coordinated course of care.

Does the government regulate chiropractic?

Chiropractic practice is regulated individually by each state and the District of Columbia. Most states require chiropractors to earn continuing education credits to maintain their licenses. Chiropractors' scope of practice varies by state, including with regard to laboratory tests or diagnostic procedures, the dispensing or selling of dietary supplements, and the use of other CAM therapies such as acupuncture or homeopathy. Chiropractors are not licensed in any state to perform major surgery or prescribe drugs.

Do health insurance plans pay for chiropractic treatment?

Compared with CAM therapies as a whole (few of which are reimbursed), coverage of chiropractic by insurance plans is extensive. As of 2002, more than 50 percent of health maintenance organizations (HMOs), more than 75 percent of private health care plans, and all state workers' compensation systems covered chiropractic treatment. Chiropractors can bill Medicare, and over two dozen states cover chiropractic treatment under Medicaid.

If you have health insurance, check whether chiropractic care is covered before you seek treatment. Your plan may require care to be approved in advance, limit the number of visits covered, and/or require that you use chiropractors within its network.

What has scientific research found out about whether chiropractic works for low-back pain?

The results of individual clinical trials and reviews of groups of clinical trials were examined. Chiropractic techniques were identified as chiropractic manipulation rather than some other forms of manipulation or spinal manipulation therapy, which may be delivered by certain other health care providers.

So far, the scientific research on chiropractic and low-back pain has focused on if, and how well, chiropractic care helps in relieving pain and other symptoms that people have with low-back pain. This research often compares chiropractic to other treatments.

Detailed findings from seven controlled clinical trials and one prospective observational study of chiropractic treatment for low-back pain published between January 1994 and June 2003 indicate at least some benefit to the participants from chiropractic treatment. However, in six of the eight studies, chiropractic and conventional treatments were found to be similar in effectiveness. One trial found greater improvement in the chiropractic group than in groups receiving either sham manipulation or back school. Another trial found treatment at a chiropractic clinic to be more effective than outpatient hospital treatment.

♣ **It's A Fact!!**

Examples Of Non-Manual Chiropractic Treatments

Heat and ice

Ultrasound

Electrical stimulation

Rehabilitative exercise

Magnetic therapy

Counseling about diet, weight loss, and other lifestyle factors

Dietary supplements

Homeopathy

Acupuncture

✎ What's It Mean?

Acupuncture: A health care practice that originated in traditional Chinese medicine. Acupuncture involves inserting needles at specific points on the body in the belief that this will help improve the flow of the body's energy (or qi, pronounced "chee") and thereby help the body achieve and maintain health.

Cauda equina syndrome: A syndrome that occurs when the nerves of the cauda equina (a bundle of spinal nerves extending beyond the end of the spinal cord) are compressed and damaged. Symptoms include leg weakness, loss of bowel, bladder, and/or sexual functions, and changes in sensation around the rectum or genitalia.

Clinical trial: A clinical trial is a research study in which a treatment or therapy is tested in people to see whether it is safe and effective. Clinical trials are a key part of the process in finding out which treatments work, which do not, and why. Clinical trial results also contribute new knowledge about diseases and medical conditions.

Controlled clinical trial: A clinical study that includes a comparison (control) group. The comparison group receives a placebo, another treatment, or no treatment at all.

General review: An analysis in which information from various studies is summarized and evaluated; conclusions are made based on this evidence.

Homeopathy: Also known as homeopathic medicine, it is an alternative medical system. In homeopathic treatment, there is a belief that "like cures like," meaning that small, highly diluted quantities of medicinal substances are given to cure symptoms, when the same substances given at higher or more concentrated doses would actually cause those symptoms.

Meta-analysis: A type of research review that uses statistical techniques to analyze results from a collection of individual studies.

Naturopathic medicine: Also known as naturopathy. It is an alternative medical system in which practitioners work with natural healing forces within the body with a goal of helping the body heal from disease and attain better health. Practices may include dietary modifications, massage, exercise, acupuncture, minor surgery, and various other interventions.

Observational study: A type of study in which individuals are observed or certain outcomes are measured. No attempt is made to affect the outcome (for example, no treatment is given).

Orthopedist: Doctor of Medicine (M.D.) who is a surgeon specializing in disorders of the musculoskeletal system.

Osteopathic medicine: Also known as osteopathy. It is a form of conventional medicine that, in part, emphasizes diseases arising in the musculoskeletal system. There is an underlying belief that all of the body's systems work together, and disturbances in one system may affect function elsewhere in the body. Most osteopathic physicians practice osteopathic manipulation, a full-body system of hands-on techniques to alleviate pain, restore function, and promote health and well-being.

Osteoporosis: A reduction in the amount of bone mass, which can lead to breaking a bone after a minor injury, such as a fall.

Placebo: Resembles a treatment being studied in a clinical trial, except that the placebo is inactive. One example is a sugar pill. By giving one group of participants a placebo and the other group the active treatment, the researchers can compare how the two groups respond and get a truer picture of the active treatment's effects. In recent years, the definition of placebo has been expanded to include other things that could affect the results of health care, such as how a patient feels about receiving the care and what he or she expects to happen from it.

Sham: A treatment or device that is a type of placebo. An example would be positioning the patient's body and placing the chiropractor's hands in a way that mimics an actual treatment, but is not a treatment.

Systematic review: A type of research review in which data from a set of studies on a particular question or topic are collected, analyzed, and critically reviewed.

Three reviews of clinical trials on chiropractic treatment for back pain published between October 1996 and June 2003 indicate the evidence was seen as weak and less than convincing for the effectiveness of chiropractic for back pain. Specifically, the 1996 systematic review reported that there were major quality problems in the studies analyzed; for example, statistics could not be effectively combined because of missing and poor-quality data. The review concludes that the data "did not provide convincing evidence for the effectiveness of chiropractic. The 2003 general review states that since the 1996 systematic review, emerging trial data "have not tended to be encouraging... The effectiveness of chiropractic spinal manipulation for back pain is thus at best uncertain. The 2003 meta-analysis found spinal manipulation to be more effective than sham therapy but no more or no less effective than other treatments.

Several other points are helpful to keep in mind about the research findings. Many clinical trials of chiropractic analyze the effects of chiropractic manipulation alone, but chiropractic practice includes more than manipulation. Results of a trial performed in one setting (such as a managed care organization or a chiropractic college) may not completely apply in other settings. And, researchers have observed that the placebo effect may be at work in chiropractic care, as in other forms of health care.

Are there scientific controversies associated with chiropractic?

Yes, there are scientific controversies about chiropractic, both inside and outside the profession. For example, within the profession, there have been disagreements about the use of physical therapy techniques, which techniques are most appropriate for certain conditions, and the concept of subluxations. Outside views have questioned the effectiveness of chiropractic treatments, their scientific basis, and the potential risks in subsets of patients (for example, the risks of certain types of adjustments to patients with osteoporosis or risk factors for osteoporosis, compared to patients with healthier bone structures).

Research studies on chiropractic are ongoing. The results are expected to expand scientific understanding of chiropractic. A key area of research is the basic science of what happens in the body (including its cells and nerves) when specific chiropractic treatments are given.

Is the National Center for Complementary and Alternative Medicine (NCCAM) funding research on chiropractic?

Yes. For example, recent projects supported by NCCAM include the following:

- Comparing conventional medical care for acute back pain with an "expanded benefits" package (consisting of conventional care plus a choice of chiropractic, massage, or acupuncture)

- Finding out what happens (through measurement) in the lumbar portion of the spine after chiropractic positioning and adjustment

- Evaluating the effects of the speed of spinal adjustment on muscles and nerves

- Studying the effectiveness of chiropractic adjustment for a variety of conditions, including neck pain, chronic pelvic pain, and temporomandibular disorders (TMD) in the jaw

Chapter 18

Craniosacral Therapy

How does craniosacral therapy (CST) work?

Craniosacral therapy works by helping the body's natural healing mechanisms dissipate the negative effects of stress on the central nervous system.

This is accomplished through utilizing a physiological body system called the craniosacral system, which maintains the environment in which the central nervous system functions. It consists of the membranes and cerebrospinal fluid that surround and protect the brain and spinal cord, extending from the bones of the skull, face, and mouth (which make up the cranium) down to the tailbone area (or sacrum). The role of this system in the development and performance of the brain and spinal cord is so vital that an imbalance or dysfunction in it can cause sensory, motor, and/or neurological disabilities.

Like the pulse of the cardiovascular system, the craniosacral system has a rhythm that can be felt throughout the body. Using a touch generally no heavier than the weight of a nickel, skilled practitioners can monitor this rhythm at key body points to pinpoint the source of an obstruction or stress.

About This Chapter: Information in this chapter is from "Frequently Asked Questions about CranioSacral Therapy." © 2006 The Upledger Clinic and The Upledger Institute, Inc. All rights reserved. Reprinted with permission.

Once a source has been determined, they can assist the natural movement of the fluid and related soft tissue to help the body self-correct. This simple action is often all it takes to remove a restriction. Other times, CST may be combined with other complementary therapies to help restore the body to its optimum functioning level.

What conditions can craniosacral therapy help?

Among CST's largest patient groups are those suffering chronic symptoms that haven't been aided by other approaches. In particular, CST is beneficial to those with head, neck, or back injuries resulting from an accident—be it from a car, sports, or work mishap, or from a fall. The extremely light touch involved in the application of CST makes it a safe approach as well for children, infants, and newborns with early traumas, including birth trauma. They especially can benefit from the timely identification and release of restrictions in the craniosacral system, thereby preventing future difficulties such as learning disabilities or hyperactivity.

♣ **It's A Fact!!**

Because of its influence on the functioning of the central nervous system, craniosacral therapy can benefit the body in a number of ways—from bolstering overall health and resistance to disease to alleviating a wide range of specific medical conditions.

Another area of principal effectiveness is with stress-related dysfunctions. Insomnia, fatigue, headaches, poor digestion, anxiety, and temporomandibular joint (TMJ) dysfunction are just a few examples. Craniosacral therapy works to reverse the debilitating effects of stress by providing the conditions in which the nervous system can rest and rejuvenate. In fact, it's this capacity to reduce stress that's leading an increasing number of people to include CST as part of their wellness routines.

Other conditions for which craniosacral therapy has shown to be effective are various sensory disorders. Among these are eye-motor coordination problems, autism, dyslexia, loss of taste or smell, tinnitus, vertigo, and neuralgias such as sciatica and tic douloureux.

Is there any condition for which CST shouldn't be used?

There are certain situations where application of CST would not be recommended. These include conditions where a variation and/or slight increase in intracranial pressure would cause instability. Acute aneurysm, cerebral hemorrhage, or other preexisting severe bleeding disorders are examples of conditions that could be affected by small intracranial pressure changes.

How many craniosacral therapy sessions will I need?

Response to CST varies from individual to individual and condition to condition. Your response is uniquely your own and can't be compared to anyone else's—even those cases that may appear to be similar to your own. The number of sessions needed varies widely—from just one up to three or more a week over the course of several weeks.

When was craniosacral therapy developed?

It was in 1970, during a neck surgery in which he was assisting, that osteopathic physician John E. Upledger first observed the rhythmic movement of what would soon be identified as the craniosacral system. None of his colleagues, or any of the medical texts at the time, could explain this discovery, however.

His curiosity piqued, Dr. Upledger began searching for the answer. He started with the research of Dr. William Sutherland, the father of cranial osteopathy. For some 20 years beginning in the early 1900s, Sutherland had explored the concept that the bones of the skull were structured to allow for movement. For decades after, this theory remained at odds with the beliefs of the scientific and medical communities. Dr. Upledger believed, however, that if Sutherland's theory of cranial movement was in fact true, this would help explain, and make feasible, the existence of the rhythm he had encountered in surgery.

It was at this point that Dr. Upledger set out to scientifically confirm the existence of cranial bone motion. From 1975 to 1983 he served as clinical researcher and Professor of Biomechanics at Michigan State University, where he supervised a team of anatomists, physiologists, biophysicists, and bioengineers in research and testing. The results not only confirmed Sutherland's theory, but also led to clarification of the mechanisms behind this motion—the craniosacral system. Dr. Upledger's continued work in the field ultimately resulted in his development of craniosacral therapy.

What is The Upledger Institute?

The Upledger Institute is a health resource center located in Palm Beach Gardens, Florida, that's recognized worldwide for its groundbreaking continuing education programs, clinical research, and therapeutic services.

The Institute was founded in 1985 by Dr. Upledger to educate the public and healthcare practitioners about the benefits of craniosacral therapy. It conducts hundreds of workshops throughout the world each year, educating healthcare practitioners of many diverse disciplines in CST. To date, more than 50,000 have been trained. Among them are osteopaths, medical doctors, doctors of chiropractic, doctors of Oriental medicine, naturopathic physicians, psychiatric specialists, psychologists, dentists, nurses, physical therapists, occupational therapists, acupuncturists, massage therapists, and other professional body workers.

Chapter 19

Hydrotherapy

What is hydrotherapy?

Hydrotherapy is the use of water to maintain health or promote healing. Ice, steam, and hot, tepid, and cold water are all used in a number of different ways—some widely accepted, others controversial. For example, external treatments, such as the application of ice to a sprained ankle or soaking in a hot tub to soothe sore muscles, have become common remedies, and both conventional and alternative practitioners, particularly naturopaths, universally prescribe some of these remedies.

Water has been part of the therapeutic arsenal since the beginning of civilization. The ancient Greek physician, Hippocrates, promoted the healthful effects of taking a bath. Regular trips to the bathhouse were part of the Roman regimen for good health and hygiene. The most rapid growth of hydrotherapy, however, occurred in Germany during the nineteenth century, when Vincenz Priessnitz (1799–1851) and Father Sebastian Kneipp (1821–1897) established independent hydrotherapy centers there.

Although many in the scientific community questioned the effects of hydrotherapy, its popularity spread. By the late-nineteenth century, hydrotherapy centers had begun to spring up in the United States in places like

Saratoga Springs, New York, Hot Springs, Arkansas, and Warm Springs, Georgia. Seeking cures for everything from arthritis to warts, wealthy visitors came regularly to these early spas to "take the waters."

❖ It's A Fact!!

Most mainstream doctors consider internal therapies, such as colonic irrigation, suspect and even dangerous.

Hydrotherapy gained some scientific credence in 1900, when J. H. Kellogg, a medical doctor and the brother of the founder of the cereal empire, published his book *Rational Hydrotherapy*. Documenting Kellogg's numerous research experiments on the therapeutic effects of water, the book quickly became the definitive work on the subject. It is still used today by many naturopaths, who learn hydrotherapy as part of their training.

How does it work?

The basic properties of water allow this nontoxic and readily available substance to be used in many aspects of patient care. Not only does water keep people hydrated, its universal solvent properties make it essential for cleaning wounds and preventing infection. Water is also useful in its other physical states: Steam can open clogged sinuses; ice packs can relieve swelling.

Hydrotherapy also takes advantage of water's unique ability to store and transmit both cold and heat. Cold-based hydrotherapies, such as ice packs and cold compresses, have what is known as a "depressant" effect: Cold decreases normal activity, constricting blood vessels, numbing nerves, and slowing respiration. On the other hand, heat-based hydrotherapies, such as whirlpools and hot compresses, have the opposite effect. As the body attempts to throw off the excess heat and keep body temperature from rising, dilation of blood vessels occurs, providing increased circulation to the area being treated.

Contrast hydrotherapies, which typically involve compresses or immersion, alternate heat with cold and are mainly used to dramatically stimulate local circulation. For example, a 30-minute contrast bath to the lower extremities (four minutes hot, one minute cold, repeated for a total of 30 minutes) can produce a 95% increase in local blood flow.

What can I expect?

Today hydrotherapy is a part of the physical therapy department of virtually every hospital and medical center. Various techniques using water are considered standard strategies for rehabilitation and relief of pain. Exercises in hydrotherapy pools, whirlpool baths, and swimming pools are among the basic offerings that continue to be a part of the long heritage of hydrotherapeutic techniques.

Some treatments are done only by a complementary care specialist, such as a naturopathic doctor; others require the supervision of a trained therapist. After examining you and taking your history, the doctor will explain how you can perform the appropriate therapy for your condition yourself or will send you to an appropriate facility.

Treatments such as icing, hot and cold compresses, friction rubs, and sitz baths are easily learned and can be done at home as part of a self-care program.

✔ **Quick Tip**

Many forms of hydrotherapy are also available at health spas and resorts. Be sure to check the credentials of the spa before going.

What are the health benefits?

Used mainly to treat wounds and burns, to provide pain relief, to facilitate physical rehabilitation, and to promote relaxation, water-based therapies are currently used throughout conventional, complementary, and alternative medicine.

The physiological effects depend on the type of hydrotherapy used. The following are commonly recommended techniques:

Icing: Ideal for strains, sprains, and bruises, icing can easily be done at home if the injury isn't too severe. If you sprain your ankle while jogging, for example, the best thing you can do is go right home and ice it to minimize the swelling and internal bleeding. Be sure to wrap the ice, whether it's ice cubes in a plastic bag or a gel pack, in a towel. Putting ice directly on your skin can cause nerve damage. Keep the ice in place for 20 minutes. Depending on the severity of the injury, repeat the ice application every two hours for 24 hours. After this time, taking a hot shower or bath, or applying a hot compress, can increase circulation to the injured area and speed the healing process.

Compresses: To make a compress, a cloth is soaked in hot or cold water and then wrung out so the desired amount of moisture remains. Single or double compresses may be used. A single compress simply involves placing one layer of the wet cloth over the affected area. A double compress involves putting a dry material such as wool or flannel over the wet compress. When using hot water, the double compress serves to retain the heat. When using cold water, the body gradually warms the compress and the transition from cold to warm adds to the therapeutic value. A cold compress can be used to prevent or relieve congestion, reduce blood flow to an area, and inhibit inflammation. A hot compress can have an analgesic effect, thereby decreasing pain. Hot compresses can also be used to lessen the discomfort from menstrual cramps and irritable bowel syndrome, and to increase blood flow to a particular part of the body. A hot or cold compress (depending on individual preference) can relieve a headache.

Baths: You can use baths to either immerse the entire body or simply the affected body part. Hot full-immersion baths can help with arthritic discomfort and conditions where muscles are in painful spasm, such as fibromyalgia. For a neutral (or tepid) bath the temperature should be neither too hot nor too cold. These are mainly used for relaxation purposes and to treat stress-related ailments such as insomnia, anxiety, and nervous exhaustion. Cool baths can relieve irritation and itching caused by hives or other skin disorders.

Sitz baths: Taking sitz baths involves partially immersing the pelvic region. A hot sitz bath can help reduce pain from hemorrhoids, menstrual cramps, and sciatica. A neutral sitz bath is best for bladder infections or severe itching in the anal region. A cold sitz bath constricts blood vessels and may be helpful for excess vaginal bleeding and mild constipation. A contrast sitz bath, from hot to cold, increases circulation in the pelvis and may be useful for chronic prostatitis and pelvic infections. You can buy a special sitz bath seat to fit over your toilet seat or you can simply sit in your bathtub.

Cold friction rubs: A friction rub involves massaging a particular area of the body with a rough washcloth, terry towel, or loofah that has first been placed in ice water. Friction rubs have a tonifying effect on the body, increasing circulation and tightening muscles.

How do I choose a practitioner?

The type of practitioner you consult depends on the nature of your ailment. If you have a sports injury, for example, you would most likely visit your primary care physician, a chiropractor, or a physical therapist. If you have a more serious condition, such as irritable bowel syndrome, you would most likely see your regular doctor or a gastroenterologist.

If you are interested in complementary forms of hydrotherapy, you might wish to talk to a licensed naturopathic doctor. To find one who practices hydrotherapy, contact a professional association.

What precautions should I take with hydrotherapy?

Take precautions with both hot and cold water treatments. Do not use a microwave to heat a compress because the material will get too hot too quickly. Soak the compress in hot water from the tap and test its temperature before applying it to your body. When using ice, do not put the ice or ice pack directly on your skin. Wrap it in a towel and then apply.

Hydrotherapy that uses extreme temperatures is not recommended for pregnant women or for people who have a heart condition, circulation disorder, high blood pressure, or diabetes.

Visit http://www.wholehealthchicago.com for more information.

Reprinted from http://www.WholeHealthChicago.com.

Chapter 20

Massage Therapy

What is massage therapy?

Many physicians have been recommending massage therapy for years—nearly 2,400 years. The Greek physician Hippocrates first documented the medical benefits of "friction" in Western culture around 400 B.C. Today, massage therapy is being used as a means of treating painful ailments, decompressing tired and overworked muscles, reducing stress, rehabilitating sports injuries, and promoting general health. This is accomplished by manipulating a client's soft tissues in order to improve the body's circulation and remove waste products from the muscles.

While massage therapy is done for medical benefit, a massage can be given to simply relax or rejuvenate the person being massaged. It is important to note that this type of massage is not intended for a medical purpose, and provides medical value only through general stress reduction and increased energy levels. Thoroughly trained individuals who provide specialized care with their client's medical health in mind, on the other hand, practice massage therapy.

Most massage therapists specialize in several modalities, which require different techniques. Some use exaggerated strokes ranging the length of a

About This Chapter: Information in this chapter is excerpted from "Massage Therapists," *Occupational Outlook Handbook, 2006-2007 Edition*, Bureau of Labor Statistics, U.S. Department of Labor, December 2005.

body part, while others use quick, percussion-like strokes with a cupped or closed hand. A massage can be as long as two hours or as short as five or ten minutes. Usually, the type of massage therapists give depends on the client's needs and the client's physical condition. For example, they use special techniques for elderly clients that they would not use for athletes, and they would use approaches for clients with injuries that would not be appropriate for clients seeking relaxation. There are also some forms of massage that are given solely to one type of client, for example prenatal massage and infant massage.

Massage therapists work by appointment. Before beginning a massage therapy session, therapists conduct an informal interview with the client to find out about the person's medical history and desired results from the massage. This gives therapists a chance to discuss which techniques could be beneficial to the client and which could be harmful. Because massage therapists tend to specialize in only a few areas of massage, customers will often be referred, or seek a therapist with a certain type of massage in mind. Based on the person's goals, ailments, medical history, and stress- or pain-related problem areas, a massage therapist will conclude whether a massage would be harmful, and if not, move forward with the session while concentrating on any areas of particular discomfort to the client. While giving the massage, therapists alter their approach or concentrate on a particular area as necessary.

Many modalities of massage therapy use massage oils, lotions, or creams to massage and rub the client's muscles. Most massage therapists, particularly those who are self-employed, supply their own table or chair, sheets, pillows, and body lotions or oils. Most modalities of massage require clients to be covered in a sheet or blanket and require clients to be undressed or to wear loose-fitting clothing. The therapist only exposes the body part on which he or she is currently massaging. Some types of massage are done without oils or lotions and are performed with the client fully clothed.

Massage can be a delicate issue for some clients, and those clients may indicate that they are comfortable with contact only in specified areas. For this reason, and also for general-purpose business risks, about half of all massage therapists have liability insurance, either through a professional association membership or through other insurance carriers.

✤ **It's A Fact!!**

Massage therapists can specialize in over 80 different types of massage, called modalities. Swedish massage, deep tissue massage, reflexology, acupressure, sports massage, and neuromuscular massage are just a few of the many approaches to massage therapy.

Massage therapists must develop a rapport with their clients if repeat customers are to be secured. Because those who seek a therapist tend to make regular visits, developing a loyal clientele is an important part of becoming successful.

What is the typical environment when getting a massage?

Massage therapists work in an array of settings both private and public: private offices, studios, hospitals, nursing homes, fitness centers, sports medicine facilities, airports, and shopping malls, for example. Some massage therapists also travel to clients' homes or offices to provide a massage. It is not uncommon for full-time massage therapists to divide their time among several different settings, depending on the clients and locations scheduled.

Most massage therapists give massages in dimly lit settings. Using candles and/or incense is not uncommon. Ambient or other calm, soothing music is often played. The dim lighting, smells, and background noise are meant to put clients at ease. On the other hand, when visiting a client's office, a massage therapist may not have those amenities. The environment depends heavily on a therapist's location and what the client wants.

What are the training standards and requirements for massage therapists?

Training standards and requirements for massage therapists vary greatly by state and locality. In 2004, 33 states and the District of Columbia had passed laws regulating massage therapy in some way. Most of the boards governing massage therapy in these states require practicing massage therapists to complete a formal education program and pass the national certification examination or a state exam. Some state regulations require that therapists keep up on their knowledge and technique through continuing education. It is best to check information on licensing, certification, and accreditation on a state-by-state basis.

Chapter 21

Reflexology

What is reflexology?

Reflexology is a complementary therapy that works on the feet or hands enabling the body to heal itself. Following illness, stress, injury, or disease, it is in a state of "imbalance" and vital energy pathways are blocked, preventing the body from functioning effectively. Reflexology can be used to restore and maintain the body's natural equilibrium and encourage healing.

A reflexologist uses hands only to apply pressure to the feet. For each person, the application and the effect of the therapy are unique. Sensitive, trained hands can detect tiny deposits and imbalances in the feet, and by working on these points the reflexologist can release blockages and restore the free flow of energy to the whole body. Tensions are eased, and circulation and elimination is improved. This gentle therapy encourages the body to heal itself, often counteracting a lifetime of misuse.

Who can benefit from reflexology?

Reflexology is suitable for all ages and may bring relief from a wide range of acute and chronic conditions. After completing a course of reflexology treatment for a specific condition, many people find it beneficial to continue with regular treatments in order to maintain health and well-being.

About This Chapter: Information in this chapter is from "About Reflexology" and "Frequently Asked Questions." Reprinted with permission from the Association of Reflexologists, http://www.aor.org.uk, © 2005. All Rights Reserved.

While many people use reflexology as a way of relaxing the mind and body and counteracting stress, at the same time, many doctors, consultants, and other health care professionals recognize reflexology as a well-established, respected, and effective therapy.

With ever increasing levels of stress, it is important people take more responsibility for their own health care needs. Reflexology helps us to cope on a physical, mental, and emotional level, thereby encouraging us to heal and maintain health in all areas of our lives.

How can reflexology help me?

Reflexology can be used to help restore and maintain the body's natural equilibrium. This gentle therapy encourages the body to work naturally to restore its own healthy balance.

Reflexology has been shown to be effective for the following:

- Back pain

- Migraine

- Infertility

- Arthritis

- Sleep disorders

- Hormonal imbalances

- Sports injuries

- Stress-related conditions

Reflexology does not claim to cure, diagnose or prescribe.

✤ It's A Fact!!
History Of Reflexology

In 1913, Dr. William Fitzgerald noted that pressure on specific parts of the body could have an anesthetizing effect on a related area. Developing this theory, he divided the body into ten equal and vertical zones, ending in the fingers and toes. He concluded that pressure on one part of a zone could affect everything else within that zone.

In the 1930s, Eunice Ingham, a therapist, further developed and refined the zone therapy into what is now known as reflexology. She observed that congestion or tension in any part of the foot mirrors congestion or tension in a corresponding part of the body. Thus, when you treat the big toes there is a related effect in the head, and treating the whole foot can have a relaxing and healing effect on the whole body.

What happens when you go for treatment?

On your first visit there is a preliminary talk with the practitioner. The reflexologist then begins to work on your feet, or hands if necessary, noting problem areas. There may be discomfort in some places, but it is fleeting, and is an indication of congestion or imbalance in a corresponding part of the body. For the most part, the sensation is pleasant and soothing.

Usually a treatment session lasts between 30 minutes to 1 hour. A course of treatment varies in length depending on your body's needs. Your reflexologist will discuss this with you at the first session.

After the first treatment or two your body may respond in a very definite way. You may have a feeling of well-being and relaxation; or you may feel lethargic, nauseous or tearful, but this is transitory. It is, however, vital information for reflexologists, as it shows how your body is responding to treatment.

Please ensure that your practitioner is professionally qualified.

Why does it hurt when I am having a treatment and what does this mean?

Reflexology can, at times, be uncomfortable. If you experience any discomfort, it is important that you inform your reflexologist on each and every occasion, as this response to the treatment helps them to build an understanding of how your body is working. Discomfort can be an indication that there is an upset in the energy flow in a particular part of the body. The point of discomfort often corresponds to an area in the body, which may be out of balance or not working as well as it could be. Often, this does not mean that there is something physically wrong with the body; rather it can give an indication of the cause behind a problem. For example, if you are visiting a reflexologist to help with back pain, you may find areas of discomfort not only in the spine reflexes but also in other areas that correspond to the spine physically, or which give an indication as to why you are suffering from a bad back in the first place. Every individual is unique in this respect and your reflexologist will discuss the patterns that emerge from each session with you.

Can reflexology have an affect on any medications I am taking?

Reflexology works by helping the body function at an optimal level. There are some circumstances where this may mean that you do not need as high a dose of medication as you would when not using reflexology. However, any change in dosage or frequency of medication must always be discussed with your doctor prior to altering medication. Contrary to popular belief, reflexology cannot "flush the system" of medication.

Chapter 22

Rolfing

Rolfing® structural integration is named after Dr. Ida P. Rolf. She began her inquiry more than fifty years ago, devoting her energy to creating a holistic system of soft tissue manipulation and movement education that organized the whole body in gravity.

Dr. Rolf discovered that she could achieve remarkable changes in posture and structure by manipulating the body's myofascial system. While she first named this work structural integration, "Rolfing" is the name that many clients and practitioners use to describe it. Rolfing is now a registered service mark in 27 countries.

Rolfing structural integration has an unequaled and unprecedented ability to dramatically alter a person's posture and structure. Professional athletes, dancers, children, business professionals, indeed people from all walks of life have benefited from Rolfing. They seek out Rolfing as a way to ease pain and chronic stress, plus improve performance in their professional and daily life activities. It's estimated that more than one million people have received Rolfing work.

Research shows that Rolfing significantly reduces chronic stress and changes in the body structure. For example, a study showed that Rolfing significantly

About This Chapter: Information in this chapter is from "Rolfing® Structural Integration," "How Rolfing Works," "Rolf Movement," and "Rolfing and Massage," accessed January 20, 2006. © The Rolf Institute® of Structural Integration. All rights reserved. Reprinted with permission. For additional information, visit http://www.rolf.org.

reduced the spinal curvature of subjects with lordosis (sway back); it also showed that Rolfing enhances neurological functioning.

How Rolfing Works

The Rolf Institute of Structural Integration (RISI) has continued Dr. Rolf's profound inquiry into how to enhance the whole person by organizing the body in gravity. Some of the more important developments of the work since Dr. Rolf's death are also what now distinguishes Rolfing from all other forms of structural integration. Some of these developments are as follows:

♣ It's A Fact!!

Research has demonstrated that Rolfing creates a more efficient use of the muscles, allows the body to conserve energy, and creates more economical and refined patterns of movement.

Source: "Rolfing® Structural Integration," © The Rolf Institute® of Structural Integration.

- **Principles of Intervention:** Rolfing training begins with the Ten Series developed by Dr. Rolf, plus variations of her original protocol. Over the years, the faculty at the Rolf Institute has articulated the core principles on which the original series was based. By understanding these principles, Rolfers can work effectively outside of the Ten Series and incorporate intervention strategies that reflect the unique needs of each client.

- **Gentle Techniques:** Rolfers work with the deep myofascial structures. Some people may experience the work as uncomfortable. Rolfers have continued to develop a broad range of techniques that produce profound results with less discomfort.

- **Joint Mobilization Techniques:** The Rolf Institute faculty has created a range of soft tissue techniques that release the motion restrictions that impede whole body organization. These techniques increase Rolfers' effectiveness in working with many common structural problems.

- **The Personal Experience:** Rolfing is a holistic technique in that changes in structure can impact the whole person, physically, emotionally, and energetically. Ultimately, each client's individual experience plays a central role in Rolfing's transformational aspects.

- **The Integration of Structure and Function:** In Rolf Movement Integration, the Rolfer helps clients become aware of their inhibiting movement patterns and teaches them how to change them. In Rolfing structural integration, the Rolfer releases these patterns through manipulation as they manifest in the client's structure. Rolfing is as concerned with how people experience and use their bodies in their daily lives as with their structural organization in gravity. This unique blend of both the functional and structural aspects of Rolfing is a distinctive feature of the training at RISI.

Rolf Movement

Towards the end of her life, Dr. Rolf believed that a movement training component would be a valuable adjunct to the structural Ten Series. Dr. Rolf collaborated first with Dorothy Nolte and then Judith Aston to develop this aspect of Rolfing. Since Dr. Rolf's death in 1979, others, including Jane Harrington, Heather Starsong, Gael Ohlgren and Vivian Jaye have elevated this less familiar style of Rolfing to a level of high art with tremendous transformative value. Currently, approximately 25% of all Rolfers have been certified in Rolf Movement and employ this training as a way of enriching their work.

The purpose of Rolf Movement is to work with the client to identify the movement patterns that promote strain and asymmetry in her system. Once these patterns are identified, the Rolf Movement practitioner doesn't necessarily seek to change those patterns, which have served the client well. Rather the Rolfer offers more economical solutions, ones that promote greater balance and efficiency in the gravitational field.

Like the structural Ten Series, Rolf Movement is taught as a sequence of sessions devoted to specific structural and movement themes. In a classic movement series, the first session is devoted to exploring breathing patterns and using the breath to promote ease and release holdings in the ribs, lungs, and respiratory diaphragm. Subsequent sessions address movement patterns in the foot, ankle and knee joints, the hip joint, the arms, and head and neck. These sessions are normally repeated to access deeper holding patterns and achieve higher levels of order just as structural Rolfers return to the extremities and upper and lower girdles (the shoulder and pelvis) in the latter sessions to more fully integrate structure and function.

While Rolf Movement can be explored by clients who have completed a structural series, it serves equally well as a stand-alone tool for achieving higher levels of self-awareness and body coherence.

Rolfing And Massage

What is the difference between massage and Rolfing? One of the most common misconceptions about Rolfing is that it is nothing more than a type of very deep massage. There are many varieties of massage, which are particularly effective for loosening tight tissue, reducing stress, detoxing the body, and increasing the feeling of relaxation and well-being. Since these benefits are also a byproduct of Rolfing, the general public experiences confusion as to the precise difference between Rolfing and the proliferation of effective touch modalities currently available. Ray McCall, an Advanced Rolfer in Boulder and former student of Dr. Rolf, once said that what Rolfers do can be summed up in three words: palpation, discrimination, and integration. They palpate, or touch the tissue, feeling for imbalances in tissue texture, quality, and temperature to determine where they need to work. They discriminate, or separate fascial layers that adhere and muscles that have been pulled out of position by strain or injury. Finally, they integrate the body, relating its segments in an improved relationship, bringing physical balance in the gravitational field. Other soft-tissue manipulation methods, including massage, are quite good at the first two, but do not balance the body in gravity. As Dr. Rolf used to say, "Anyone can take a body apart, very few know how to put it back together." The true genius of her method is the art and science of reshaping and reorganizing human structure according to clearly defined principles in a systematic and consistent manner.

In addition their skill as structural integrators, they are also educators, a point Dr. Rolf stressed frequently in her training classes. The role of teacher is something every Rolfer takes seriously. In each session, Rolfers seek to impart insights to clients to increase their awareness and understanding, to help the client make the work they do their own. Their job is to make themselves obsolete, by empowering their clients to take charge of their own physical and emotional health. Influencing the structural evolution of man on a global level was Dr. Rolf's fondest dream.

Part Four

Dietary And Herbal Remedies

Chapter 23

Dietary Supplements

Questions And Answers About Dietary Supplements

Dietary supplements are a topic of great public interest. Whether you are in a store, using the internet, or talking to people you know, you may hear about supplements and claims of benefits for health. How do you find out whether what's in the bottle is safe to take and whether science has proven that the product does what it claims? This chapter provides some answers.

What are dietary supplements?

Dietary supplements (also called nutritional supplements, or supplements for short) were defined in a law passed by Congress in 1994. They are defined as follows:

- They are taken by mouth.

- They contain a "dietary ingredient" intended to supplement the diet. Examples of dietary ingredients include vitamins, minerals, herbs (as single herbs or mixtures), other botanicals, amino acids, and dietary substances such as enzymes and glandulars.

About This Chapter: This chapter begins with "Questions And Answers About Dietary Supplements" excerpted from "What's in the Bottle? An Introduction to Dietary Supplements," National Center for Complementary and Alternative Medicine (NCCAM), National Institutes of Health, NCCAM Publication No. D191, July 2004. Text under the heading "Tips For The Savvy Supplement User" is excerpted from *FDA Consumer*, U.S. Food and Drug Administration, March-April 2002.

- They come in different forms, such as tablets, capsules, soft gels, gel caps, liquids, and powders.

- They are not represented for use as a conventional food or as a sole item of a meal or the diet.

- They are labeled as being a dietary supplement.

Dietary supplements are sold in grocery, health food, drug, and discount stores, as well as through mail order catalogs, TV programs, the internet, and direct sales.

Is using supplements considered conventional medicine or complementary and alternative medicine (CAM)?

Some uses of dietary supplements have become part of conventional medicine. For example, scientists have found that the vitamin folic acid prevents certain birth defects, and a regimen of vitamins and zinc can slow the progression of the eye disease age-related macular degeneration.

On the other hand, some supplements are considered to be complementary and alternative medicine (CAM)—either the supplement itself or one or more of its uses. An example of a CAM supplement would be an herbal formula that claims to relieve arthritis pain but has not been proven to do so through scientific studies. An example of a CAM use of a supplement would be taking 1,000 milligrams of vitamin C per day to prevent or treat a cold, as the use of large amounts of vitamin C for these purposes has not been proven.

How can I get science-based information on a supplement?

There are several ways to get information on supplements that is based on the results of rigorous scientific testing, rather than on testimonials and other unscientific information.

- Ask your health care provider. Even if your provider does not happen to know about a particular supplement, he can access the latest medical guidance about its uses and risks.

- Dietitians and pharmacists also have helpful information.

- You can find out yourself whether there are any scientific research findings on the complementary and alternative medicine (CAM)

supplement you are interested in. The National Center for Complementary and Alternative Medicine (NCCAM) and other federal agencies have free publications, clearinghouses, and databases with this information.

If I am interested in using a supplement as CAM, how can I do so most safely?

Here are some points to keep in mind:

- It is important to talk to your health care provider (or providers, if you have more than one) about the supplement. This is for your safety and a complete treatment plan. It is especially important to talk to your provider if the following is true:

  - You are thinking about replacing your regular medical care with one or more supplements.

  - You are taking any medications (whether prescription or over-the-counter). Some supplements have been found to interact with medications.

  - You have a chronic medical condition.

  - You are planning to have surgery. Certain supplements may in-crease the risk of bleeding or affect anesthetics and painkillers.

- Do not take a higher dose of a supplement than what is listed on the label, unless your health care provider advises you to do so.

- If you experience any side effects that concern you, stop taking the supplement and contact your provider. You can also report your expe-rience to the U.S. Food and Drug Administration's (FDA) Med Watch program, which tracks consumer safety reports on supplements.

- For current information from the federal government on the safety of particular supplements, check the "Alerts and Advisories" section of the NCCAM website (http://ncam.nih.gov/health/allerts) or the FDA's Center for Food Safety and Applied Nutrition "Warnings and Safety Information" website (http://www.cfsan.fda.gov/%7edms/ds-warn.html).

I see the word "natural" on a lot of supplement labels. Does "natural" always mean "safe"?

There are many supplements, as well as many prescription drugs, that come from natural sources and are both useful and safe. However, "natural" does not always mean "safe" or "without harmful effects." For example, consider mushrooms that grow in the wild—some are safe to eat, while others are poisonous.

The FDA issues warnings about supplements that pose risks to consumers, including those used for CAM therapies.

Does the federal government regulate supplements?

Yes, the federal government regulates supplements through the FDA. Currently, the FDA regulates supplements as foods rather than drugs. In general, the laws about putting foods (including supplements) on the market and keeping them on the market are less strict than the laws for drugs. Here are the specifics:

♣ It's A Fact!!
Supplements And Drugs Can Interact

- St. John's wort can increase the effects of prescription drugs used to treat depression. It can also interfere with drugs used to treat HIV infection, to treat cancer, for birth control, or to prevent the body from rejecting transplanted organs.

- Ginseng can increase the stimulant effects of caffeine (as in coffee, tea, and cola). It can also lower blood sugar levels, creating the possibility of problems when used with diabetes drugs.

- Ginkgo, taken with anticoagulant or antiplatelet drugs, can increase the risk of bleeding. It is also possible that ginkgo might interact with certain psychiatric drugs and with certain drugs that affect blood sugar levels.

Source: National Center for Complementary and Alternative Medicine.

- Research studies in people to prove a supplement's safety are not required before the supplement is marketed, unlike for drugs.

- The manufacturer does not have to prove that the supplement is effective, unlike for drugs. The manufacturer can say that the product addresses a nutrient deficiency, supports health, or reduces the risk of developing a health problem, if that is true. If the manufacturer does make a claim, it must be followed by the statement "This statement has not been evaluated by the Food and Drug Administration. This product is not intended to diagnose, treat, cure, or prevent any disease."

- The manufacturer does not have to prove supplement quality. These are the specifics:

  - The FDA does not analyze the content of dietary supplements.

  - At this time, supplement manufacturers must meet the requirements of the FDA's Good Manufacturing Practices (GMPs) for foods. GMPs describe conditions under which products must be prepared, packed, and stored. Food GMPs do not always cover all issues of supplement quality. Some manufacturers voluntarily follow the FDA's GMPs for drugs, which are stricter.

  - Some manufacturers use the term "standardized" to describe efforts to make their products consistent. However, U.S. law does not define standardization. Therefore, the use of this term (or similar terms such as "verified" or "certified") does not guarantee product quality or consistency.

- If the FDA finds a supplement to be unsafe once it is on the market, only then can it take action against the manufacturer and/or distributor, such as by issuing a warning or requiring the product to be removed from the marketplace.

The federal government also regulates supplement advertising through the Federal Trade Commission. It requires that all information about supplements be truthful and not mislead consumers.

♣ It's A Fact!!
Ephedra Ban: No Shortage of Reasons

The Food and Drug Administration (FDA) has banned the sale of dietary supplements containing ephedra (ephedrine alkaloids) due to concerns over their cardiovascular effects, including increased blood pressure and irregular heart rhythm. The final rule, published February 6, 2004, became effective on April 12, 2004.

"This FDA rule reflects what the scientific evidence shows—that ephedra poses an unreasonable risk to those who use it," the Health and Human Services Secretary said. "The regulations prohibit the sale of dietary supplements containing ephedra, and we intend to take swift action against anyone who puts consumers at risk by continuing to sell such products after the prohibition takes effect."

The action banning ephedra, often referred to as ma huang, marks the first time that the FDA has taken formal action to halt the sale of a dietary supplement ingredient since passage of the Dietary Supplement Health and Education Act (DSHEA) in 1994.

Ephedra is a naturally occurring substance found in plants. Its principal active ingredient is ephedrine, an amphetamine-like compound that potentially has powerful stimulant effects on the nervous system and heart. Like an amphetamine, ephedra increases both blood pressure and heart rate, decreases appetite, and makes the user feel energetic.

In synthetic form, ephedrine is regulated as a drug under the Federal Food, Drug and Cosmetic Act (FD&C Act), and is allowed as an ingredient in over-the-counter drugs to treat asthma, nasal congestion, and minor eye irritation. In recent years, however, dietary supplement products containing botanical ephedra, often in combination with caffeine, another type of stimulant, have been promoted to help people lose weight and enhance sports performance and energy. At the same time, ephedra has been suspected of causing unreasonable health risks or injuries.

Evidence Of Harm

There is strong scientific evidence of harm associated with the use of ephedra products. The FDA has been reviewing information for many years about ephedra's effects in the body, its safety and effectiveness, and the adverse event reports associated with its use. The agency found that supplements containing ephedra show little evidence of effectiveness, except for short-term weight loss. The agency also found that the herbal substance raises blood pressure and stresses the circulatory system. These reactions have been linked to serious health problems, including heart ailments and strokes.

One review sponsored by the National Institutes of Health concluded that ephedra is associated with higher risks of mild-to-moderate heart palpitations, psychiatric and upper gastrointestinal effects, and symptoms of hyperactivity of the autonomic nervous system, such as tremor and insomnia, especially when taken with caffeine and other stimulants. Another review showed that, for people taking more than 32 milligrams daily, the rate of hemorrhagic (bleeding) strokes among ephedra users was significantly higher than that recorded for non-users. Some ephedra-containing dietary supplement labels recommend daily doses of up to 100 milligrams.

Additionally, a study of calls to poison control centers revealed a disproportionate rate of reactions to ephedra relative to other herbal products. In short, the evidence shows that ephedra is associated with an increased risk of alarming side effects, possibly even deaths.

Products Affected By The Ban

All currently marketed dietary supplements are affected by the ban if they contain a source of ephedrine alkaloids, including the following:

- Ephedra

- Ma huang

- *Sida cordifolia*

- Pinellia

The rule does not pertain to the following:

- Traditional Chinese herbal remedies

- Herbal teas regulated as conventional foods subject to FDA regulation under other sections of the law

- Drugs that contain chemically synthesized ephedrine

Source: U.S. Food and Drug Administration, *FDA Consumer*, March-April 2004.

Is NCCAM supporting research on supplements?

Yes, NCCAM is funding most of the nation's current research aimed at increasing scientific knowledge about supplements including whether they work; if so, how they work; and how purer and more standardized products could be developed. The following is a list of some substances that researchers are studying:

- Yeast-fermented rice, to see if it can lower cholesterol levels in the blood

- Soy, to see if it slows the growth of tumors

- Ginger and turmeric, to see if they can reduce inflammation associated with arthritis and asthma

- Chromium, to better understand its biological effects and impact upon insulin in the body, possibly offering new pathways to treating type 2 diabetes

- Green tea, to find out if it can prevent heart disease

NCCAM is also sponsoring or cosponsoring clinical trials on supplements, including the following:

- Glucosamine hydrochloride and chondroitin sulfate, to find out if they relieve knee pain from osteoarthritis

- Black cohosh, to see if it reduces hot flashes and other symptoms of menopause

- Echinacea, to see if it shortens the length or lessens the severity of colds in children

---

♣ It's A Fact!!

What's In The Bottle Does Not Always Match What's On The Label

- A supplement might not contain the correct ingredient (plant species). For example, one study that analyzed 59 preparations of echinacea found that about half did not contain the species listed on the label.

- A supplement might contain higher or lower amounts of the active ingredient. For example, an NCCAM-funded study of ginseng products found that most contained less than half the amount of ginseng listed on their labels.

- A supplement might be contaminated.

Source: National Center for Complementary and Alternative Medicine.

- Garlic, to find out if it can lower moderately high cholesterol levels

- Ginkgo biloba, to determine whether it prevents or delays decline in cognitive (thinking) function in people aged 85 or older

- Ginger, to confirm whether it eases nausea and vomiting after cancer chemotherapy

Tips For The Savvy Supplement User

Think about your total diet. Dietary supplements are intended to supplement the diets of some people, but not to replace the balance of the variety of foods important to a healthy diet. While you need enough nutrients, too much of some nutrients can cause problems.

Ask yourself: Does it sound too good to be true? Do the claims for the product seem exaggerated or unrealistic? Are there simplistic conclusions being drawn from a complex study to sell a product? While the internet can be a valuable source of accurate, reliable information, it also has a wealth of misinformation that may not be obvious. Learn to distinguish hype from evidence-based science. Nonsensical lingo can sound very convincing. Also, be skeptical about anecdotal information from persons who have no formal training in nutrition or botanicals, or personal testimonials (from store employees, friends, or online chat rooms and message boards) about incredible benefits or results obtained from using a product. Question these people on their training and knowledge in nutrition or medicine.

Think twice about chasing the latest headline. Sound health advice is generally based on a body of research, not a single study. Be wary of results claiming a "quick fix" that depart from previous research and scientific beliefs. Keep in mind science does not proceed by dramatic breakthroughs, but by taking many small steps, slowly building towards a consensus. Furthermore, news stories about the latest scientific study, especially those on TV or radio, are often too brief to include important details that may apply to you or allow you to make an informed decision.

Check your assumptions about the following:

Questionable Assumption #1—"Even if a product may not help me, it at least won't hurt me." It is best not to assume that this will always be true. When consumed in high enough amounts, for a long enough time, or in combination with certain other substances, all chemicals can be toxic, including nutrients, plant components, and other biologically active ingredients.

Questionable Assumption #2—"When I see the term 'natural,' it means that a product is healthful and safe." Consumers can be misled if they assume this term assures wholesomeness, or that these food-like substances necessarily have milder effects, which makes them safer to use than drugs. The term "natural" on labels is not well defined and is sometimes used ambiguously to imply unsubstantiated benefits or safety. For example, many weight-loss products claim to be "natural" or "herbal" but this does not necessarily make them safe. Their ingredients may interact with drugs or may be dangerous for people with certain medical conditions.

Questionable Assumption #3—"A product is safe when there is no cautionary information on the product label." Dietary supplement manufacturers may not necessarily include warnings about potential adverse effects on the labels of their products. If consumers want to know about the safety of a specific dietary supplement, they should contact the manufacturer of that brand directly. It is the manufacturer's responsibility to determine that the supplement it produces or distributes is safe and that there is substantiated evidence that the label claims are truthful and not misleading.

✎ What's It Mean?

Amino acid: Building block of proteins.

Botanical: See "herb." "Botanical" is a synonym for "herb."

Enzymes: Proteins that speed up chemical reactions in the body.

Glandulars: Dietary ingredients or supplements that are made from the glands of animals.

Herb: A plant or plant part that is used for its flavor, scent, and/or therapeutic properties.

Source: National Center for Complementary and Alternative Medicine.

Questionable Assumption #4—"A recall of a harmful product guarantees that all such harmful products will be immediately and completely removed from the marketplace." A product recall of a dietary supplement is voluntary and, while many manufacturers do their best, a recall does not necessarily remove all harmful products from the marketplace.

Contact the manufacturer for more information about the specific product that you are purchasing. If you cannot tell whether the product you are purchasing meets the same standards as those used in the research studies you read about, check with the manufacturer or distributor. Ask to speak to someone who can address your questions, some of which may include the following:

1. What information does the firm have to substantiate the claims made for the product? Be aware that sometimes firms supply so-called "proof" of their claims by citing undocumented reports from satisfied consumers, or "internal" graphs and charts that could be mistaken for evidence-based research.

2. Does the firm have information to share about tests it has conducted on the safety or efficacy of the ingredients in the product?

3. Does the firm have a quality control system in place to determine if the product actually contains what is stated on the label and is free of contaminants?

4. Has the firm received any adverse event reports from consumers using their products?

Chapter 24

Botanical Supplements

What is a botanical?

A botanical is a plant or plant part valued for its medicinal or therapeutic properties, flavor, and/or scent. Herbs are a subset of botanicals. Products made from botanicals that are used to maintain or improve health may be called herbal products, botanical products, or phytomedicines.

Can botanicals be dietary supplements?

To be classified as a dietary supplement, a botanical must meet the following definition.

As defined by Congress in the Dietary Supplement Health and Education Act, which became law in 1994, a dietary supplement is a product (other than tobacco) that meets the following criteria:

• It is intended to supplement the diet.

• It contains one or more dietary ingredients (including vitamins, minerals, herbs or other botanicals, amino acids, and other substances) or their constituents.

• It is intended to be taken by mouth as a pill, capsule, tablet, or liquid.

About This Chapter: Information in this chapter is excerpted from "Botanical Dietary Supplements: Background Information," Office of Dietary Supplements, National Institutes of Health, July 2004.

- It is labeled on the front panel as being a dietary supplement.

Many botanical preparations meet this definition.

How are botanicals commonly sold and prepared?

Botanicals are sold in many forms such as fresh or dried products, liquid or solid extracts, tablets, capsules, powders, and tea bags. For example, fresh ginger root is often found in the produce section of food stores; dried ginger root is sold packaged in tea bags, capsules, or tablets; and liquid preparations made from ginger root are also sold. A particular group of chemicals or a single chemical may be isolated from a botanical and sold as a dietary supplement, usually in tablet or capsule form. An example is phytoestrogens from soy products.

Common preparations include teas, decoctions, tinctures, and extracts:

- A tea, also known as an infusion, is made by adding boiling water to fresh or dried botanicals and steeping them. The tea may be drunk either hot or cold.

- Some roots, bark, and berries require more forceful treatment to extract their desired ingredients. They are simmered in boiling water for longer periods than teas, making a decoction, which also may be drunk hot or cold.

- A tincture is made by soaking a botanical in a solution of alcohol and water. Tinctures are sold as liquids and are used for concentrating and preserving a botanical. They are made in different strengths that are expressed as botanical-to-extract ratios (i.e., ratios of the weight of the dried botanical to the volume or weight of the finished product).

- An extract is made by soaking the botanical in a liquid that removes specific types of chemicals. The liquid can be used as is or evaporated to make a dry extract for use in capsules or tablets.

Are botanical dietary supplements standardized?

Standardization is a process that manufacturers may use to ensure batch-to-batch consistency of their products. In some cases, standardization involves identifying specific chemicals (also known as markers) that can be

♣ It's A Fact!!
Dandelion

What It Is Used For

- Dandelion has been used in many traditional medical systems, including Native American and traditional Arabic medicine.

- Historically, dandelion was most commonly used to treat liver diseases, kidney diseases, and spleen problems. Less commonly, dandelion was used to treat digestive problems and skin conditions.

- Today, dandelion is used by some as a liver or kidney "tonic," as a diuretic, and for minor digestive problems.

How It Is Used

The leaves and roots of the dandelion, or the whole plant, are used fresh or dried in teas, capsules, or extracts. Dandelion leaves are used in salads or as a cooked green, and the flowers are used to make wine.

What The Science Says

There is no compelling scientific evidence for using dandelion as a treatment for any medical condition.

Side Effects And Cautions

- Dandelion use is generally considered safe. However, there have been rare reports of upset stomach and diarrhea, and some people are allergic to the plant.

- People with an inflamed or infected gallbladder, or blocked bile ducts, should avoid using dandelion.

- It is important to inform your health care providers about any herb or dietary supplement you are using, including dandelion. This helps to ensure safe and coordinated care.

Source: National Center for Complementary and Alternative Medicine (NCCAM), National Institutes of Health, NCCAM Publication No. D302, January 2006.

used to manufacture a consistent product. The standardization process can also provide a measure of quality control.

Dietary supplements are not required to be standardized in the United States. In fact, no legal or regulatory definition exists for standardization in the United States as it applies to botanical dietary supplements. Because of this, the term "standardization" may mean many different things. Some

---

✔ Quick Tip
Consider Safety When Using Herbal Supplements

1. It's important to know that just because an herbal supplement is labeled "natural" does not mean it is safe or without any harmful effects. For example, the herbs kava and comfrey have been linked to serious liver damage.

2. Herbal supplements can act in the same way as drugs. Therefore, they can cause medical problems if not used correctly or if taken in large amounts. In some cases, people have experienced negative effects even though they followed the instructions on a supplement label.

3. Women who are pregnant or nursing should be especially cautious about using herbal supplements, since these products can act like drugs. This caution also applies to treating children with herbal supplements.

4. It is important to consult your health care provider before using an herbal supplement, especially if you are taking any medications (whether prescription or over-the-counter). Some herbal supplements are known to interact with medications in ways that cause health problems. Even if your provider does not know about a particular supplement, he can access the latest medical guidance on its uses, risks, and interactions.

5. If you use herbal supplements, it is best to do so under the guidance of a medical professional who has been properly trained in herbal medicine. This is especially important for herbs that are part of an alternative medical system, such as the traditional medicines of China, Japan, or India.

6. In the United States, herbal and other dietary supplements are regulated by the U.S. Food and Drug Administration (FDA) as foods. This means that they do not have to meet the same standards as drugs and over-the-counter

manufacturers use the term standardization incorrectly to refer to uniform manufacturing practices; following a recipe is not sufficient for a product to be called standardized. Therefore, the presence of the word "standardized" on a supplement label does not necessarily indicate product quality.

Ideally, the chemical markers chosen for standardization would also be the compounds that are responsible for a botanical's effect in the body. In

medications for proof of safety, effectiveness, and what the FDA calls Good Manufacturing Practices.

7. The active ingredient(s) in many herbs and herbal supplements are not known. There may be dozens, even hundreds, of such compounds in an herbal supplement. Scientists are currently working to identify these ingredients and analyze products using sophisticated technology. Identifying the active ingredients in herbs and understanding how herbs affect the body are important research areas for the National Center for Complementary and Alternative Medicine.

8. Published analyses of herbal supplements have found differences between what's listed on the label and what's in the bottle. This means that you may be taking less, or more, of the supplement than what the label indicates. Also, the word "standardized" on a product label is no guarantee of higher product quality, since in the United States there is no legal definition of "standardized" (or "certified" or "verified") for supplements.

9. Some herbal supplements have been found to be contaminated with metals, unlabeled prescription drugs, microorganisms, or other substances.

10. There has been an increase in the number of websites that sell and promote herbal supplements on the internet. The federal government has taken legal action against a number of company sites because they have been shown to contain incorrect statements and to be deceptive to consumers. It is important to know how to evaluate the claims that are made for supplements.

Source: "Herbal Supplements: Consider Safety, Too" National Center for Complementary and Alternative Medicine (NCCAM), National Institutes of Health, NCCAM Publication No. D190, September 2004.

this way, each lot of the product would have a consistent health effect. However, the components responsible for the effects of most botanicals have not been identified or clearly defined.

Are botanical dietary supplements safe?

Many people believe that products labeled "natural" are safe and good for them. This is not necessarily true because the safety of a botanical depends on many things, such as its chemical makeup, how it works in the body, how it is prepared, and the dose used.

The action of botanicals range from mild to powerful (potent). A botanical with mild action may have subtle effects. Chamomile and peppermint, both mild botanicals, are usually taken as teas to aid digestion and are generally considered safe for self-administration. Some mild botanicals may have to be taken for weeks or months before their full effects are achieved. For example, valerian may be effective as a sleep aid after 14 days of use but it is rarely effective after just one dose. In contrast a powerful botanical produces a fast result. Kava, as one example, is reported to have an immediate and powerful action affecting anxiety and muscle relaxation.

The dose and form of a botanical preparation also play important roles in its safety. Teas, tinctures, and extracts have different strengths. The same amount of a botanical may be contained in a cup of tea, a few teaspoons of tincture, or an even smaller quantity of an extract. Also, different preparations vary in the relative amounts and concentrations of chemical removed from the whole botanical. For example, peppermint tea is generally considered safe to drink but peppermint oil is much more concentrated and can be toxic if used incorrectly. It is important to follow the manufacturer's suggested directions for using a botanical and not exceed the recommended dose without the advice of a health care provider.

Does a label indicate the quality of a botanical dietary supplement product?

It is difficult to determine the quality of a botanical dietary supplement product from its label. The degree of quality control depends on the manufacturer, the supplier, and others in the production process.

The U.S. Food and Drug Administration (FDA) is authorized to issue Good Manufacturing Practice (GMP) regulations describing conditions under which dietary supplements must be prepared, packed, and stored. Some manufacturers voluntarily follow drug GMPs, which are more rigorous, and some organizations that represent the dietary supplement industry have developed unofficial GMPs.

What methods are used to evaluate the health benefits and safety of a botanical dietary supplement?

Scientists use several approaches to evaluate botanical dietary supplements for their potential health benefits and safety risks, including their history of use and laboratory studies using cell or animal models. Studies involving people (individual case reports, observational studies, and clinical trials) can provide information that is relevant to how botanical dietary supplements are used. Researchers may conduct a systematic review to summarize and evaluate a group of clinical trials that meet certain criteria. A meta-analysis is a review that includes a statistical analysis of data combined from many studies.

Chapter 25

Detox Diets

The name sounds reassuring—everyone knows that anything toxic is bad for you. Plus these diets encourage you to eat natural foods and involve lots of water and veggies—all stuff you know is good for you. You hear about celebrities going on detox diets, and people who go into drug or alcohol rehabs are said to be detoxing. So shouldn't a detox diet be a good bet?

Not really. Like many other fad diets, detox diets can have harmful side effects, especially for teens.

First, let's look at the lingo. A toxin is a chemical or poison that is known to have harmful effects on the body. Toxins can come from food or water, from chemicals used to grow or prepare food, and even from the air that we breathe. Our bodies bring in toxins and then process those toxins through organs like the liver and kidneys and eliminate them in the form of sweat, urine, and feces.

What is a detox diet?

The people who support detox diets say that because of emotional stress or dehydration, toxins don't leave our bodies properly during the elimination

About This Chapter: Information in this chapter is from "Are Detox Diets Safe?" This information was provided by TeensHealth, one of the largest resources online for medically reviewed health information written for parents, kids, and teens. For more articles like this one, visit www.TeensHealth.org, or www.KidsHealth.org. © 2003 The Nemours Center for Children's Health Media, a division of The Nemours Foundation.

of waste. Instead, they believe toxins hang around in our digestive, lymph, and gastrointestinal systems as well as in our skin and hair. According to proponents of detox diets, these toxins can cause all kinds of problems, like tiredness, headaches, nausea, and acne.

So the basic idea behind detox diets is to temporarily give up certain kinds of foods that are thought to contain toxins. The idea is to purify and purge your body of all the "bad" stuff. Although the diets vary, most of them involve some version of a fast, that is, giving up food for a couple of days, and then gradually reintroducing certain foods into your diet. Many of these diets also encourage you to undergo colonic irrigation, otherwise known as an enema (an enema flushes out your rectum and colon using water), which is designed to "clean out" your colon. Still others recommend that you take herbal supplements to help the "purification" process.

There are tons of detox diets out there. Typically they involve 1 or 2 days on a completely liquid diet and another 4 or 5 days adding brown rice, fruit, and steamed vegetables (all organic) to the diet. After a week of eating only these foods, you gradually reintroduce other foods—except for red meat, wheat, sugar, eggs, and all prepackaged or junk foods—into your diet.

People on detox diets are also encouraged to chew their food thoroughly, to drink very little while eating, and to relax prior to each meal (although it seems a stretch to call a glass of lemon water a meal!).

Lots of claims are made about what a detox diet can do for you, from preventing and curing disease to giving you more energy to making you

✎ What's It Mean?

Colonic Irrigation: Another term for enema. [1]

Enema: The injection of a liquid through the anus into the large bowel. [2]

Laxative: A substance that promotes bowel movements. [2]

Toxin: A poison produced by certain animals, plants, or bacteria. [2]

Source: [1] Editor. [2] "Dictionary of Cancer Terms," National Cancer Institute, U.S. National Institutes of Health, cited July 2006.

more focused and clear-headed. Of course, anyone who goes on a low-fat, high-fiber diet is probably going to feel more healthy, but proponents of detox diets claim that this is because of the elimination of toxins, as opposed to carrying around less excess weight or having a healthier heart. However, there's no scientific proof that these diets help rid the body of toxins faster or that the elimination of toxins will make you a healthier, more energetic person.

What should you watch out for?

If detox diets still appeal to you, there are a couple of things you should keep in mind. For starters, detox diets are intended for short-term purposes only. (People are usually encouraged to go on fasts like this at specific times during the year, such as at the end of a season.) And these diets are usually recommended not to help people lose weight, but to help clean out their systems.

Because normal teenagers need lots of good nutrition, with high calories and protein to support the teenage growth and development period, diets that involve fasting and severe restriction of food are not a good idea. For teens who are involved in sports and physical activities that require ample food, fasting does not provide enough fuel to support these activities. For these reasons, detox diets can be especially risky for teenagers.

It's not recommended that people with diabetes, low blood sugar, or eating disorders go on detox diets.

You should also know that this type of diet can be addicting—some people really like purging. That's because there's a certain feeling that comes from going without food or having an enema—almost like the high other people get from nicotine or alcohol. This purification buzz can become a dangerous addiction that leads to health problems, including serious eating disorders and even death.

In addition, many of the supplements called for by these diets are actually laxatives, which are designed to make you go to the bathroom more often. These types of supplements are never a good idea because they can cause dehydration, mineral imbalances, and problems with your digestive system.

Finally, if you fast for several days, you may drop pounds but most of it will be water and some of it may be muscle, which will make you look thin and flabby, rather than tight and toned. Fasting for longer periods can also slow down your metabolism, making it harder to keep the weight off or to lose weight later.

We're not going to tell you that eating lots of veggies and fiber and drinking lots of water is a bad idea. But you also need to make sure you're getting all of the nutrients you need, including protein from lean meats, eggs, beans, or peas and calcium from low-fat or fat-free milk or yogurt. You definitely shouldn't start a detox diet or stop eating from any major food group without talking to your doctor or a registered dietitian.

Your body is designed to purify itself. Your liver and kidneys will do the job they're supposed to do if you eat a healthy diet that includes fiber, fruits, veggies, and plenty of water. If you're feeling tired or run down, or if you're concerned that you're overweight, talk with a doctor who can help you determine the cause and recommend ways to address the problem.

Chapter 26

Macrobiotic Diet

The word "macrobiotic" comes from Greek roots and means "long life". A Japanese educator named George Ohsawa, who believed that simplicity was the key to optimal health, developed the macrobiotic diet and philosophy. The diet Ohsawa recommended included ten progressively restrictive stages. The last stage of Ohsawa's macrobiotic diet consisted only of brown rice and water. Due to its extreme restriction, macrobiotic diet counselors no longer recommend Ohsawa's version of the macrobiotic diet.

Michio Kushi expanded on Ohsawa's macrobiotic theory and opened the Kushi Institute in Boston in 1978. Together with his wife Aveline, Kushi published many books on macrobiotics and was responsible for popularizing the diet in North America.

Why do people follow this diet?

People seeking a healthy way of eating that integrates physical, spiritual, and planetary health are interested in the macrobiotic diet. The macrobiotic diet is a low-fat, high-fiber diet that is a predominantly vegetarian diet, emphasizing whole grains and vegetables. In addition, the macrobiotic diet is rich in phytoestrogens from soy products.

About This Chapter: Information in this chapter is from "The Macrobiotic Diet," © 2006 by Cathy Wong (http://altmedicine.about.com/od/popularhealthdiets/a/Macrobiotic.htm). Used with permission of About, Inc., which can be found online at www.about.com. All rights reserved.

Because low-fat, high-fiber diets are often recommended for cancer and other chronic diseases, the macrobiotic diet has been used by people with these conditions. The phytoestrogen content may be protective and reduce the risk of estrogen-related cancers such as breast cancer. However, further research is needed to clarify whether the macrobiotic diet is effective in cancer prevention and treatment.

What are the guidelines of this diet?

- **Whole grains—50–60% of each meal:** Whole grains include brown rice, whole wheat berries, barley, millet, rye, corn, buckwheat, and other whole grains. Rolled oats, noodles, pasta, bread, baked goods, and other flour products can be eaten occasionally.

> **♣ It's A Fact!!**
> People with serious medical conditions, such as cancer or AIDS, should always seek proper medical care. Some people try the diet because they heard it can cure their disease, but research has not substantiated these claims.

- **Soup—1 to 2 cups or bowls of soup per day:** Miso and shoyu, which are made from fermented soybeans, are commonly used.

- **Vegetables—25–30% of daily food intake:** Up to one-third of the total vegetable intake can be raw. Otherwise, vegetables should be steamed, boiled, baked, and sautéed.

- **Beans—10% of daily food intake:** Cooked beans or bean products such as tofu, tempeh, and natto.

- **Animal Food—Small amount of fish or seafood several times per week. Avoid meat, poultry, eggs, and dairy:** Consume with horseradish, wasabi, ginger, mustard, or grated daikon to help the body detoxify from the effects of fish and seafood.

- **Seeds and Nuts—In moderation:** Seeds and nuts can be lightly roasted and salted with sea salt or shoyu.

- **Local Fruit—Several times a week:** Apples, pears, peaches, apricots, grapes, berries, melons, and other fruit. Avoid tropical fruit such as mango, pineapple, and papaya.

- **Desserts—In moderation, 2–3 times per week:** Desserts can be enjoyed by people who are in good health. Emphasize naturally sweet foods such as apples, squashes, adzuki beans, and dried fruit. Natural sweeteners such as rice syrup, barley malt, and amazake can be used. Avoid sugar, honey, molasses, chocolate, carob, and other sweeteners.

- **Cooking Oil—Use unrefined vegetable oil:** The most common is dark sesame oil. Other oils that are recommended are light sesame oil, corn oil, and mustard seed oil.

- **Condiments and Seasonings:** Commonly used seasonings include natural sea salt, shoyu, brown rice vinegar, umeboshi vinegar, umeboshi plums, grated ginger root, fermented pickles, gomashio (roasted sesame seeds), roasted seaweed, and sliced scallions.

Diet guidelines should be individualized based on factors such as climate, season, age, gender, activity, and health needs.

What are the strengths of this diet?

This diet emphasizes the foods that tend to be lacking in the North American diet—fiber-rich whole grains, vegetables, and beans. It is low in saturated fat and high in phytoestrogens, which may help to balance women's hormones and help with menopause, premenstrual syndrome, and prevention against breast cancer and endometriosis.

In addition, the macrobiotic diet is low in meat, dairy products, and sugar.

Are there any possible complications or side effects of this diet?

The macrobiotic diet is considered by some nutritionists to be too restrictive and lacking in certain nutrients, such as protein, vitamin B_{12}, iron, magnesium, and calcium. Lack of energy may result from inadequate protein.

Chapter 27

Raw Food Diet

The raw food diet has become popular recently, thanks to high-profile adherents like actor Woody Harrelson, model Carol Alt, designer Donna Karan, and Chicago-based celebrity chef Charlie Trotter.

What is the raw food diet?

The raw food diet is based on unprocessed and uncooked plant foods, such as fresh fruits and vegetables, sprouts, seeds, nuts, grains, beans, nuts, dried fruit, and seaweed.

Heating food above 116 degrees Fahrenheit is believed to destroy enzymes in food that can assist in the digestion and absorption of food. Cooking is also thought to diminish the nutritional value and "life force" of food.

At least 75 percent of the diet must be living or raw.

What are the benefits of the raw food diet?

Proponents of the raw food diet believe it has numerous health benefits, including the following:

- Increased energy
- Improved skin appearance
- Better digestion
- Weight loss
- Reduced risk of heart disease

The raw food diet contains little or no saturated fat and trans fats. It is also low in sodium, high in potassium, magnesium, folate, fiber, and health-promoting plant chemicals called phytochemicals.

These properties are associated with a reduced risk of diseases such as heart disease, diabetes, and cancer.

For example, a study published in the *Journal of Nutrition* found that consumption of a raw food diet lowered plasma total cholesterol and triglyceride concentrations.

What are the guidelines of the raw food diet?

1. **What can I eat?** Eat unprocessed, preferably organic, whole foods such as the following:

   - Fresh fruits and vegetables
   - Nuts
   - Seeds
   - Beans
   - Grains
   - Legumes
   - Dried fruit
   - Seaweed
   - Unprocessed organic or natural foods
   - Freshly juiced fruit and vegetables
   - Purified water

   > ♣ **It's A Fact!!**
   > **Side Effects Of A Raw Food Diet**
   >
   > Some people experience a detoxification reaction when they start the raw food diet, especially if their previous diet was rich in meat, sugar, and caffeine. Mild headaches, nausea, and cravings can occur and usually last for several days.

- Young coconut milk

At least 3/4 of food consumed should not be heated over 116 degrees Fahrenheit.

2. **What cooking techniques are used?** Specific cooking techniques make foods more digestible and add variety to the diet. They include the following:

   - Sprouting seeds, grains, and beans
   - Juicing fruits and vegetables
   - Soaking nuts and dried fruit
   - Blending
   - Dehydrating food

3. **What equipment can I use?** The following equipment is used for preparing the food in a raw food diet:

   - A dehydrator, a piece of equipment that blows air through food at a temperature of less than 116 degrees F.
   - A good-quality juice extractor for juicing fruits and vegetables
   - A blender, food processor, or chopper to save time
   - Large glass containers to soak and sprout seeds, grains, and beans
   - Mason jars for storing sprouts and other food

What precautions should be taken?

The raw food diet may not be appropriate for certain people, such as the following:

- Children
- Pregnant or nursing women
- People with anemia
- People at risk for osteoporosis (A Washington University study found that people following a raw food diet had lower bone mass. Bone turnover rates, however, were similar to the group that ate a standard American diet.)

Considerable time, energy, and commitment are needed to be healthy on the raw food diet. Many of the foods are made from scratch. Some ingredients may be hard to find, such as Rejuvelac (the fermented liquid drained from sprouted grains), sprouted flour, date sugar, young coconut milk, carob powder, and Celtic sea salt.

People must be aware that certain nutritional deficiencies can occur on the raw food diet, which include the following:

- Calcium

- Iron

- B_{12} (The *Journal of Nutrition* study found that a raw food diet increased levels of homocysteine, due to vitamin B_{12} deficiency.)

- Protein

- Calories

Critics of the raw food diet say, while it's true that some enzymes are inactivated when food is heated, it doesn't matter because the body uses its own enzymes for digestion. In addition, cooking makes certain phytochemicals easier to absorb, such as beta-carotene in carrots.

Another critique is that the human body has changed in response to eating cooked foods. Some of these changes are that our jaws and teeth have become smaller, our stomachs have shrunk, and our small intestines have grown longer, lengthening the digestive surface area.

According to other alternative diet theories, such as macrobiotics, Ayurveda, and traditional Chinese medicine, a raw-only diet may not be appropriate for people living in colder climates or for people with certain constitutional types.

Chapter 28

Vegetarian Diets

For much of the world, vegetarianism is largely a matter of economics—meat costs a lot more than, say, beans or rice. As such, meat becomes a special occasion dish (if it's eaten at all). Even where meat is more plentiful, it's still used in moderation, often providing a side note to a meal rather than taking center stage.

In countries like the United States where meat is not as expensive, though, people choose to be vegetarians for reasons other than economics. Parental preferences, religious beliefs, lifestyle factors, and health issues are among the most common reasons for choosing to be a vegetarian. Many people choose a vegetarian diet out of concern over animal rights or the environment. And lots of people have more than one reason for choosing vegetarianism.

Vegetarian And Semi-Vegetarian Diets

Different people follow different forms of vegetarianism. A true vegetarian eats no meat at all, including chicken and fish. A lacto-ovo vegetarian eats dairy products and eggs, but excludes meat, fish, and poultry. It follows,

About This Chapter: Information in this chapter is from "Is a Vegetarian Diet Right for Me?" This information was provided by TeensHealth, one of the largest resources online for medically reviewed health information written for parents, kids, and teens. For more articles like this one, visit www.TeensHealth.org, or www.KidsHealth.org. © 2003 The Nemours Center for Children's Health Media, a division of The Nemours Foundation.

then, that a lacto vegetarian eats dairy products but not eggs, whereas an ovo vegetarian eats eggs but not dairy products.

A stricter form of vegetarianism is a vegan (pronounced: vee-gun or vee-jan) diet. Not only are eggs and dairy products excluded from a vegan diet, so are animal products like honey and gelatin. There are a surprising number of foods that you'd think might be vegetarian but aren't—foods like gelatin, which are made using meat byproducts; cheese, which is made using an animal-based product called rennet, and sauces such as Worcestershire sauce. Vegans avoid all these foods.

Some macrobiotic diets fall into the vegan category. Macrobiotic diets restrict not only animal products but also refined and processed foods, foods with preservatives, and foods that contain caffeine or other stimulants.

Following a macrobiotic or vegan diet could lead to nutritional deficiencies in teens, who need to be sure their diets include enough nutrients to fuel growth, particularly protein and calcium. If you're interested in following a vegan or macrobiotic diet, it's a good idea to talk to a registered dietitian. He or she can help you design meal plans that include adequate vitamins and minerals.

Some people consider themselves semi-vegetarians and eat fish and maybe a small amount of poultry as

---

✎ What's It Mean?

Lacto Vegetarian: A diet that consists of plant foods plus some, or all, dairy products. [1]

Lacto-Ovo Vegetarian: A diet that consists of plant foods, milk, dairy products, and eggs. [1]

Macrobiotic Diet: A low-fat, high-fiber, predominantly vegetarian diet that restricts refined and processed foods, preservatives, caffeine, and other stimulants. [2]

Ovo Vegetarian: A diet consisting of plant foods and eggs but no dairy or meat products. [2]

Pesci-Vegetarian: A diet consisting of plant foods and fish but no other meat products. [2]

Semi-Vegetarian: A diet that restricts, but does not entirely eliminate, meat and other animal products. [2]

Vegan: A diet that consists of only foods of plant origin. [1]

Source: [1] "Glossary of Terms," Division of Workplace Programs, Substance Abuse and Mental Health Services Administration, cited July 2006. [2] Editor.

part of a diet that's primarily made up of vegetables, fruits, grains, legumes, seeds, and nuts. A pesci-vegetarian eats fish, but not poultry.

Are These Diets OK For Teens?

In the past, choosing not to eat meat or animal-based foods was considered unusual in the United States. Times and attitudes have changed dramatically, however. Vegetarians are still a minority in the United States, but a large and growing one. The American Dietetic Association (ADA) has officially endorsed vegetarianism, stating "appropriately planned vegetarian diets are healthful, are nutritionally adequate, and provide health benefits in the prevention and treatment of certain diseases."

So what does this mean for you? If you're already a vegetarian, or are thinking of becoming one, it means that you're in good company. There are more choices in the supermarket than ever before, and an increasing number of restaurants and schools are providing vegetarian options—way beyond a basic peanut butter and jelly sandwich.

If you're choosing a vegetarian diet, the most important thing you can do is to educate yourself. That's why the ADA says that a vegetarian diet needs to be "appropriately planned." Simply dropping certain foods from your diet isn't the way to go if you're interested in maintaining good health, a high energy level, and strong muscles and bones.

Vegetarians have to be careful to include the following key nutrients because they may be lacking in a vegetarian diet: iron, calcium, protein, vitamins D and B_{12}, and zinc. If meat, fish, dairy products, and/or eggs are not going to be part of your diet, you'll need to know how to get enough of these nutrients, or you may need to take a daily multiple vitamin and mineral supplement.

Here are some suggestions.

Iron: Sea vegetables like nori, wakame, and dulse are very high in iron. Less exotic but still good options are iron-fortified breakfast cereals, legumes (chickpeas, lentils, and baked beans), soybeans and tofu, dried fruit (raisins and figs), pumpkin seeds, broccoli, and blackstrap molasses. Eating these foods with a food high in vitamin C (citrus fruits and juices, tomatoes, and broccoli) will help you to better absorb the iron. Girls need to be particularly concerned about getting adequate iron because some iron is lost during menstruation. Some girls who are vegetarians may not get adequate iron from vegetable sources and require a daily supplement. Check with your doctor about your own iron needs.

Calcium: Milk and yogurt are tops if you're eating dairy products; otherwise, tofu, fortified soy milk, calcium-fortified orange juice, green leafy vegetables, and dried figs are excellent choices. Remember that as a teen you're building up your bones for the rest of your life. Because women have a greater risk for getting osteoporosis (weak bones) as adults, it's particularly important for them to make sure they get enough calcium. Again, taking a supplement may be necessary to ensure this.

Vitamin D: Cow's milk and sunshine are tops on the list for this vitamin, which you need to get calcium into your bones. Vegans can try fortified soy milk and fortified breakfast cereals, but they may need a supplement that includes vitamin D, especially during the winter months. Everyone should have some exposure to the sun to help the body produce vitamin D.

Protein: Some people believe that vegetarians must combine incomplete plant proteins in one meal—like red beans and rice—to make the type of complete proteins found in meat. We now know that it's not that complicated. Current recommendations are that vegetarians eat a wide variety of foods during the course of a day. Eggs and dairy products are good sources of protein, but also try nuts, peanut butter, tofu, beans, seeds, soy milk, grains, cereals, and vegetables to get all the protein your body needs.

Vitamin B_{12}: B_{12} is an essential vitamin found only in animal products, including eggs and dairy. Fortified soy milk and fortified breakfast cereals also have this important vitamin. It's hard to get enough vitamin B_{12} in your diet if you are vegan, so a supplement may be needed.

Zinc: If you're not eating dairy foods, make sure fortified cereals, dried beans, nuts, and soy products like tofu and tempeh are part of your diet so you can meet your daily requirement for this important mineral.

In addition to vitamins and minerals, vegetarians need to keep an eye on their total intake of calories and fat. Vegetarian diets tend to be high in fiber and low in fat and calories. That may be good for people who need to lose weight or lower their cholesterol, but it can be a problem for kids and teens who are still growing and people who are already at a healthy weight. Diets that are high in fiber tend to be more filling, and as a result strict vegetarians may feel full before they've eaten enough calories to keep their bodies healthy and strong. It's a good idea to let your doctor know that you're a vegetarian so that he or she can keep an eye on your growth and make sure you're still getting adequate amounts of calories and fat.

Getting Some Guidance

When Danielle's mom knew that she was serious about becoming a vegetarian, she made an appointment for Danielle to talk with a registered dietitian. The dietitian and Danielle went over lists of foods and recipe ideas that would give her the nutrients she needs. They discussed ways to prevent conditions such as iron-deficiency anemia that Danielle might be at an increased risk of developing. And whenever Danielle sees her family doctor, the doctor reminds her to eat many different kinds of foods each day and to get enough protein and iron.

Danielle also tries to remember to take a daily standard multivitamin, just in case she's missed getting enough vitamins or minerals that day.

Tips For Eating Out

Danielle admits that eating out can be difficult sometimes, but because she does eat fish, she can usually find something suitable on a restaurant menu. If not, she opts for salad and an appetizer or two. Even fast food places sometimes have vegetarian choices, such as bean tacos and burritos, veggie burgers made from soybeans, and soy cheese pizza.

Because both she and her sister are vegetarians, Danielle's family rarely eats red meat anymore. Her mom serves salmon frequently, and Danielle eats a lot of pasta, along with plenty of vegetables, grains, and fruits. Danielle is also psyched about some of the vegetarian products now available in the grocery store. The veggie burgers, hot dogs, and chicken substitutes taste very much like the real thing. She especially likes the ground soy "beef" that makes a great stand-in for ground beef in foods like tacos and spaghetti sauce.

☞ **Remember!!**

It's important to eat a wide variety of foods, and to try out new foods, too—regardless of whether you choose a vegetarian way of life.

Part Five

Mind-Body Medicine

Chapter 29

Mind-Body Medicine: An Overview

What is mind-body medicine?

Mind-body medicine is an approach to healing that uses the power of thoughts and emotions to positively influence physical health. As Hippocrates once wrote, "The natural healing force within each one of us is the greatest force in getting well." This is the essence of mind-body medicine.

What is the history of mind-body medicine?

Most ancient healing practices, such as Traditional Chinese Medicine and Ayurvedic medicine, emphasize the important links between the mind and the body. Western medical views were shaped by systems of thought that emphasized the opposite: the mind and body are separate. As science developed, and with Louis Pasteur's discovery of germs, the notion of a connection between mind and body was thought to be superstition.

In 1964, psychiatrist George Solomon saw that rheumatoid arthritis worsened when people were depressed. This led him to investigate the impact of emotions on inflammation and immune function in general. Thus began the new field of psychoneuroimmunology ("psycho" for psychology; "neuro" for neurology, or nervous system; and "immunology" for immunity).

About This Chapter: Information in this chapter is from "Mind-Body Medicine." © 2006 A.D.A.M., Inc. Reprinted with permission.

In the 1960s and early 1970s, a physician named Herbert Benson, who coined the term "relaxation response," studied the effects of meditation on blood pressure. Further understanding of the mind-body link came in 1975 when psychologist Robert Ader showed that mental and emotional cues affect immunity.

Today, there is renewed interest in age-old traditions such as yoga and meditation. No longer viewed with suspicion, mind-body programs are now established at prestigious medical schools in the United States and around the world.

What are mind-body techniques?

The key to any mind-body technique is to "train" the mind to focus on the body without distraction. It is in this state of "focused concentration" that an individual may be able to change his or her health. The following are some of the most commonly practiced techniques.

Biofeedback: Biofeedback is a technique in which people are trained to improve their health by learning to control certain internal bodily processes that normally occur involuntarily, such as heart rate or blood pressure. These activities can be measured with electrodes and displayed on a monitor that both the participant and his or her practitioner can see. The monitor thereby provides feedback to the participant about the internal workings of his or her body. This person can then be taught to use this information to gain control over these "involuntary" activities. Biofeedback is an effective therapy for many conditions, but it is primarily used to treat tension headache, migraine headache, and chronic pain.

Cognitive behavioral therapy: This technique is used to help people recognize and change dysfunctional thought patterns. For example, people with phobias might deliberately expose themselves, under the direction and guidance of the therapist, to what they are afraid of. Brain scans show that over time this therapy can actually change how the brain functions.

Relaxation techniques: There are three major types of relaxation techniques, which are as follows:

- Autogenic training: This technique uses both visual imagery and body awareness to move a person into a deep state of relaxation. The person imagines a peaceful place and then focuses on different physical sensations, moving from the feet to the head. For example, one might focus on warmth and heaviness in the limbs; easy, natural breathing; or a calm heartbeat.

* Progressive muscle relaxation: This technique involves slowly tensing and then releasing each muscle group individually, starting with the muscles in the toes and finishing with those in the head.

* Meditation: The two most popular forms of meditation in the U.S. include Transcendental Meditation (students repeat a mantra [a single word or phrase],) and mindfulness meditation (students focus their attention on their moment-by-moment thoughts and sensations).

Hypnosis: During hypnosis (taken from the Greek term *hypnos*, meaning "sleep") a person's body relaxes while his or her thoughts become more focused and attentive. It is in this state of deep concentration that people are highly responsive to a hypnotherapist's suggestions. Today, many mental health professionals use hypnosis to treat people with addictions, pain, anxiety disorders, and phobias.

Spirituality: Many researchers have been studying how spiritual beliefs, attitudes, and practices influence health. In a recent study on people with human immunodeficiency virus (HIV), for example, people who had faith in God, compassion toward others, a sense of inner peace, and were religious, had a better chance of surviving for a long time with acquired immune deficiency syndrome (AIDS) than those who did not have such faith or practices. Research suggests that qualities like faith, hope, and forgiveness and the use of social support and prayer have a noticeable effect on health and healing.

Does mind-body medicine work?

While phrases such as "mind over matter" have been around for years, only recently have scientists found solid evidence that mind-body techniques actually do combat disease and promote health. In 1989, for example, a landmark study by David Spiegel, M.D. at Stanford University School of Medicine, dramatically demonstrated the power of the mind to heal. Of 86 women with late-stage breast cancer, half received standard medical care while the other half received the standard care plus weekly support sessions in which the women were able to share both their grief and their triumphs. Spiegel discovered that the women who participated in the social support group lived twice as long as the women who did not. A similar study in 1999 showed that in breast cancer patients, helplessness and hopelessness are linked to lesser chances of survival.

Many recent studies also document the effect of meditation on mood and symptoms in people with different types of conditions (such as high blood pressure, irritable bowel syndrome, and cancer) as well as improve quality of life.

How does mind-body medicine work?

Researchers have found that stress hormones are associated with particular unhealthy emotions. These hormones affect systems and organs throughout the body. For example, stress related to hostility and anxiety can result in disruptions in heart and immune function. Similarly, depression and distress may diminish the body's natural capacity to heal. In contrast, emotional expression that encourages openness and active coping with problems helps stabilize the immune system.

> ✢ **It's A Fact!!**
> The goal of mind-body techniques is to activate the relaxation response and reduce the stress response.

Certain emotions have been linked to disease. For example, hostile attitudes may increase your risk for coronary heart disease, obesity (particularly having excess fat around the waist), insulin resistance (which can lead to diabetes), and abnormal cholesterol (specifically, high triglycerides and low HDL— the good kind of cholesterol).

Generally, research shows that being stressed and having negative emotions is unhealthy. One study found that unconsciously being defensive or stifling feelings resulted in serious medical consequences, such as high blood pressure. High blood pressure is also associated with feelings of hopelessness. How a person processes emotions also affects how long he or she may survive a chronic illness.

The goal of mind-body techniques is to activate the relaxation response and reduce the stress response. When you are relaxed, the levels of hormones related to stress are reduced and your immune system is more efficient. High levels of stress hormones circulating in the body may actually prove to increase one's susceptibility to infection as well.

What is mind-body medicine good for?

Mind-body techniques are helpful for many conditions because they promote relaxation, improve coping skills, reduce tension and pain, and lessen the need for medication. For example, many mind-body techniques are used (along with medication) to treat acute pain. Symptoms of anxiety and depression also respond well to mind-body techniques. Because they improve coping skills and give a feeling of control over symptoms, mind-body techniques may help treat many different diseases.

In an analysis of mind-body studies, researchers found that cognitive behavioral therapy is the most long-lasting treatment for tinnitus (ringing in the ears), but relaxation techniques, hypnosis, and biofeedback were all also effective treatments. Some researchers believe that chronic fatigue syndrome, which affects the immune system, is best understood and treated with mind-body medicine.

Is there anything I should watch out for?

There is a danger that mind-body medicine might encourage you to feel that you caused your illness because you lacked a healthy mental attitude. This incorrect idea can lead to blame, and blame only causes feelings of distress and guilt.

Mind-body medicine is generally very safe and works well as an adjunct to usual medical care. Each mind-body technique may have its own risks and side effects associated with the practice. Talk with your doctor about any concerns you may have.

How can I find more information on mind-body medicine?

Biofeedback: Specialists who provide biofeedback training range from psychiatrists and psychologists to nurses, dentists, and physicians. The Association for Applied Psychology and Biofeedback (www.aapb.org) is the national membership association for professionals using biofeedback and is a good resource for finding qualified biofeedback practitioners in your area.

Relaxation: Numerous clinics and hospitals around the country have integrated relaxation techniques into their health care programs. To learn more about relaxation techniques and to locate health care facilities that include them as part of their practice, contact the Stress Reduction Clinic at the University of Massachusetts Memorial Medical Center in Worcester, Massachusetts. You can visit them on the web at www.umassmed .edu/cfm/mbsr to find a list of the health care facilities in 38 states that offer information on and training in relaxation techniques.

Hypnosis: Most hypnotherapists are licensed medical doctors, registered nurses, social workers, or family counselors that have received additional training in hypnotherapy. For example, members of the American Society of Clinical Hypnosis (ASCH) must hold a doctorate in medicine, dentistry, podiatry, or psychology, or a master's level degree in nursing, social work, psychology, or marital/family therapy with at least 20 hours of ASCH-approved training in hypnotherapy. For more information, contact either the American Society of Clinical Hypnosis (visit them on the web at www.asch.net) or the Society for Clinical and Experimental Hypnosis (on the web at www.sceh.us).

Spirituality: To learn more about spirituality's role in health (including the latest research on this topic), contact the International Center for the Integration of Health and Spirituality (visit their website at www.nihr.org).

✤ It's A Fact!!

Mind-Body Techniques May Help Treat Many Diseases

- high blood pressure
- asthma
- coronary heart disease
- obesity
- cancer, such as pain and nausea/ vomiting related to chemotherapy
- insomnia
- anxiety
- diabetes
- stomach and intestinal disorders (including indigestion [dyspepsia], irritable bowel syndrome, constipation, diarrhea, ulcerative colitis, heartburn, and Crohn disease)
- fibromyalgia
- menopausal symptoms such as hot flashes, depression, and irritability

Chapter 30

Biofeedback

What is biofeedback?

Biofeedback is a technique in which people are trained to improve their health by learning to control certain internal bodily processes that normally occur involuntarily, such as heart rate, blood pressure, muscle tension, and skin temperature. These activities can be measured with electrodes and displayed on a monitor that both the participant and his or her practitioner can see. The monitor provides feedback to the participant about the internal workings of his or her body. This person can then be taught to use this information to gain control over these "involuntary" activities. Biofeedback is an effective therapy for many conditions, but it is primarily used to treat high blood pressure, tension headache, migraine headache, chronic pain, and urinary incontinence.

Are there different types of biofeedback?

The three most commonly used forms of biofeedback therapy are the following:

- electromyography (EMG), which measures muscle tension;

- thermal biofeedback, which measures skin temperature;

About This Chapter: Information in this chapter is from "Biofeedback." © 2006 A.D.A.M., Inc. Reprinted with permission.

- neurofeedback or electroencephalography (EEG), which measures brain wave activity.

How does biofeedback work?

Scientists are not able to explain exactly how or why biofeedback works. However, there does seem to be at least one common thread: most people who benefit from biofeedback have conditions that are brought on or made worse by stress. For this reason, many scientists believe that relaxation is key to successful biofeedback therapy. When a body is repeatedly stressed, internal processes like blood pressure become overactive. Guided by a biofeedback therapist, a person can learn to lower his or her blood pressure through relaxation techniques and mental exercises. When a person successfully relaxes and lowers his or her blood pressure, the feedback signals reflect this accomplishment. This acts as affirmation and encouragement for the person's continued efforts.

What happens during a biofeedback session?

In a normal biofeedback session, electrodes are attached to the skin. These electrodes then feed information to a small monitoring box that translates the physiologic responses into a tone that varies in pitch, a visual meter that varies in brightness, or a computer screen that varies the lines moving across a grid. The biofeedback

♣ **It's A Fact!!**

Biofeedback may be useful for the following health problems:

- anorexia nervosa
- anxiety
- asthma
- autism
- back pain
- bed-wetting
- chronic pain
- constipation
- depression
- diabetes
- fecal incontinence
- epilepsy and related seizure disorders
- head injuries
- high blood pressure
- learning disabilities
- motion sickness
- muscle spasms
- sexual disorders, including pain with intercourse
- spinal cord injuries

therapist then leads the person in mental exercises. Through trial and error, people can soon learn to identify and control the mental activities that will bring about the desired physical changes.

What is biofeedback good for?

Various forms of biofeedback appear to be effective for a range of health problems. For example, biofeedback shows considerable promise for the treatment of urinary incontinence, which affects over 15 million Americans. Many people prefer biofeedback to medicine because of the lack of side effects. One early study found that biofeedback improves bladder function and reduces symptoms of urinary incontinence by up to 94 percent. Based on these and other findings, the Agency for Health Care Policy and Research has recommended biofeedback therapy as a treatment for urinary incontinence. Biofeedback also appears to be helpful for people with fecal incontinence.

Research also suggests that thermal biofeedback may soothe the symptoms of Raynaud's disease (a condition that causes diminished blood flow to fingers, toes, nose or ears) while EMG biofeedback has been shown to reduce pain, morning stiffness, and the number of tender points in people with fibromyalgia. In addition, a review of scientific studies found that biofeedback might help people with insomnia fall asleep.

In addition, one preliminary study found that the combination of temperature biofeedback and EEG neurofeedback helped alcoholics feel less depressed and more likely to abstain from drinking alcohol.

Biofeedback can also be used effectively for certain ailments in children. For example, EEG neurofeedback (especially when combined with cognitive therapy) has been shown to improve behavior and intelligence scores in children with attention deficit/hyperactivity disorder (ADHD). Biofeedback combined with fiber may also help relieve abdominal pain in children. Thermal biofeedback helps alleviate migraine and chronic tension headaches among children and adolescents as well.

How many sessions will I need?

Each session generally lasts less than one hour. The number of sessions required depends on the condition being treated. Many people begin to see results within 8 to 10 sessions. Treatment of headache, incontinence, and Raynaud's disease (as mentioned, a condition that causes diminished blood flow to the fingers, toes, nose, or ears) requires at least 10 weekly sessions and then less frequent sessions as health improves. Conditions like high blood pressure, however, usually require 20 weekly biofeedback sessions before improvement can be seen. In addition to these sessions, you will also be taught mental exercises and relaxation techniques that can be done at home and must be practiced at least 5 to 10 minutes every day.

Are there any risks associated with biofeedback?

Biofeedback is considered a safe procedure. No negative side effects have been reported.

How can I find a qualified practitioner?

Specialists who provide biofeedback training range from psychiatrists and psychologists to nurses, dentists, and physicians. The Association for Applied Psychology and Biofeedback (www.aapb.org) is the national membership association for professionals using biofeedback and is a good resource for finding qualified biofeedback practitioners in your area.

Chapter 31

Guided Imagery And Visualization

What is imagery? It's what we see or sense in our imagination. That statement alone is enough to put it in the realm of the unreal; but imagine, if you will, where the human race would be without it.

It took a great deal of imagination, that is, the ability to create new ideas, to invent the wheel, the car, a plane, or a spacecraft. Anything built, created or invented was done so using human imagination. It is not very highly valued in our culture, yet without it we would be long extinct.

The earliest visualization techniques on record are from Samaria, Babylonia, and ancient Egypt. From Hermetic rites to help a person visualize himself in perfect health, to present day pilgrims traveling to Mecca, and from the famous healing temples of ancient Greece to modern day Christian Science, visualization has been employed as a powerful tool for inner change.

According to Martin L. Rossman, M.D., "Imagery is a flow of thoughts you can see, hear, feel, smell or taste. An image is an inner representation of your experience or your fantasies—a way your mind codes, stores, and expresses information. Imagery is the currency of dreams and daydreams,

About This Chapter: "An Exploration of Guided Imagery and Visualization" by Virginia Angelou, © 2001. Reprinted with permission. Virginia Angelou is a certified teacher, practitioner & research consultant for a number of complimentary therapies.

memories and reminiscence, plans, projections, and possibilities. It is the language of
the arts, the emotions, and most important, the deeper self. Imagery is a window on your inner world—a way of
viewing your own ideas, feelings, and in-
terpretations. But it is more than just a
mere window; it is a means of transformation and liberation from distortions in this
realm that may unconsciously direct your life and shape your health."

> ♣ **It's A Fact!!**
> Many psychologists are recognizing imagery and visualization as among the most powerful tools in cognitive psychology.

Dr. Rossman goes on to say that imagery can help health concerns from a simple tension headache or a life-threatening disease.

You may be able to reduce, modify or eliminate pain, see if your lifestyle habits have contributed to your illness and decide what changes you can make to support your recovery. Imagery can help you tap inner strengths and find hope, courage, patience, perseverance, love, and other qualities that can help you cope with, transcend or recover from almost any illness.

It is refreshing to see the amount of interest being generated in the field of the mind-body connection. Imagery has been proven to have a remarkable effect on the body—affecting numerous activities including brain wave patterns, blood pressure, sexual arousal, oxygen consumption, levels of hormones in the blood, and immune system function, to name a few. In the larger context of healing, imagery can be a very effective method in aiding recovery from illness, changing relationships and lifestyle and the state of emotions by helping people to imagine what these changes need to be and how best to make them.

Guided imagery is, as its name implies, guiding a person or group with words designed to create images for various different purposes, such as relaxation, stress management, and healing—both mental and physical—and receiving information from within. These can incorporate the participation of all the senses, as explained by the following simple scenario.

Picture yourself lying under a large tree. Feel the soft warm grass with your hands. Hear the rustling of the leaves over your head. Smell the scent of aromatic flowers wafting gently on the breeze. Picture the tree overhead shading you from the sun.

To explain what is meant by imagery as opposed to visualization, Patricia Norris, Ph.D. states, "Visualization is the consciously chosen, intentional instruction to the body. Imagery is the spontaneously occurring "answer," qualifier, and modifier from the unconscious. Thus, a two-way communication is set up by the interplay of visualization and imagery. The visualization acts as a message to the unconscious. The images are messages from the unconscious to consciousness, much as dreams are.

So what is a guided imagery session like? Let's look at a basic relaxation session. Generally one person or small groups are catered for in a warm, safe, comfortable, and enclosed environment. Small groups are preferred because there are fewer chances for distractions than with larger groups. Warmth, as the climate dictates, is best since participants will usually be lying down. Mats on the floor, with pillows for support, and blankets is ideal, with space between for movement or access if anyone needs to leave. Having said this, an outdoor location can be wonderful if it is quiet, warm, and you won't be disturbed.

Lying is preferable to sitting as complete relaxation is essential. An enclosed space is more secure, and people need to feel they are safe; plus the therapist does not want to worry about interruptions. Take the phone off the hook. A "Please do not disturb" sign on the door can prevent people from walking in by accident in a more public setting.

♣ **It's A Fact!!**

Through imagery you can relax and learn to be more comfortable in any situation, whether you are ill or well.

Clothing should be loose and comfortable, and shoes removed if desired. Carefully selected music can be especially useful to create the right atmosphere and even become part of the experience. Certain natural sounds, such as birds or whales which, while soothing in the right circumstances, can be distracting from the vocal guidance. Music should enhance rather than interfere. Soft lighting is preferable, such as small lamps or carefully placed candles.

In addition, aromatherapy oils or incense can create a pleasant ambiance, but should be subtle and not overpowering. Ideally everyone should agree on the scent; if someone doesn't like a certain smell it will interfere with his or her concentration. Water and tissues should be available.

A pre-session phase is useful to give participants a brief overview of what will be happening. The session usually starts with a general relaxing exercise, such as some deep breathing and body awareness. Then the therapist may describe a more detailed visualization in which all five senses are used. At this point it should be made clear that it takes practice to imagine with all the senses; for example, some people have great difficulty seeing colors, or imagining a smell, taste, sound, or sensation.

Everyone's ability is different and must be respected. If you are new to imagery, it is perfectly fine to just "know" you are lying on a beach and the sky is blue, and to relax into that awareness. An experienced therapist will make everyone comfortable in the knowledge that their individual observations will be unique, even though the vocal guidance is the same for everyone. Trying too hard will defeat the purpose.

The main aspect of the guided imagery follows on from this, and the list of places and things that can be incorporated is endless. A common format is to guide the group to a specific location, perhaps a deserted beach, remote mountainside, lush rain forest, tranquil stream etc., and incorporate various ideas designed to make use of the senses without being too complex. Everyone will perceive and interpret these ideas differently.

No two trees will look the same, no two skies will be the same blue. Each person will have his or her own individual experience while "being surrounded by a healing white light," and every lemon will taste unique to its taster; but ultimately, the objective of relaxation will be achieved. Don't be surprised if some people fall asleep. Obviously they are in need of a rest.

The session will be far more successful if the therapist follows a few simple guidelines. The voice should enhance, not interfere with the dialogue; therefore, strong accents and the use of too flowery or infrequently used words may be distracting and should be avoided. Dialogue should be kept simple, and spoken in low tones in a pleasant, soothing, and calming voice.

Reading someone else's script can sound forced, and an experienced therapist will create the imagery so it flows naturally. Time must be allowed for people to create each image, whether visually or with the senses.

A session is brought to a close by ending the imagery and gently bringing the group's awareness back to the present time and location. A suggestion might be some deep breaths, yawning, body awareness, and gentle stretches, followed by turning on one side and slowly sitting up in their own time. Some people will want to share their personal experience while others will want to remain quiet, and the space should be held to permit a post-session phase to accommodate everyone.

A typical session may last from 15 minutes to half an hour or more, depending on content and objectives. Sessions can be attended as frequently as the client wishes. There is no known harm that can be caused by imagery, guided or otherwise, when used with positive intent. It is not to be confused with hypnosis, another very effective modality. Complete control is maintained throughout, and the recipient decides if, and to what extent, they participate.

Guided imagery practitioners come from all walks of life. Some are medically trained, and others are alternative therapists or counselors incorporating this method to compliment other treatments. It is wise to check any practitioner's credentials before embarking on a course of therapy.

Chapter 32

Hypnosis

Definition Of Hypnosis

Hypnosis is a state of inner absorption, concentration, and focused attention. It is like using a magnifying glass to focus the rays of the sun and make them more powerful. Similarly, when our minds are concentrated and focused, we are able to use our minds more powerfully. Because hypnosis allows people to use more of their potential, learning self-hypnosis is the ultimate act of self-control.

Everyone has experienced a trance many times; but we don't usually call it hypnosis. All of us have been so absorbed in thought while reading a book or riding the bus to school or work that we fail to notice what is happening around us. While we were zoned out, another level of consciousness, which we refer to as our unconscious mind, took over. These are very focused states of attention similar to hypnosis.

Clinical hypnotists do essentially three things with hypnosis. They encourage the use of imagination. Mental imagery is very powerful, especially in a focused state of attention. The mind seems capable of using imagery,

About This Chapter: Information in this chapter is from "Information for the General Public." © 2006 American Society of Clinical Hypnosis. All rights reserved. Reprinted with permission. For additional information, contact the American Society of Clinical Hypnosis, 140 North Bloomingdale Road, Bloomingdale, IL 60108, 630-980-4740, or at their website, http://www.asch.net.

even if it is only symbolic, to assist us in bringing about the things we are imagining. For example, a patient with ulcerative colitis may be asked to imagine what her distressed colon looks like. If she imagines it as being like a tunnel, with very red, inflamed walls that are rough in texture, the patient may be encouraged in hypnosis (and in self-hypnosis) to imagine this image changing to a healthy one.

Another basic hypnotic method is to present ideas or suggestions to the patient. In a state of concentrated attention, ideas and suggestions that are compatible with what the patient wants seem to have a more powerful impact on the mind.

Finally, hypnosis may be used for unconscious exploration to better understand underlying motivations or identify whether past events or experiences are associated with causing a problem. Hypnosis avoids the critical censor of the conscious mind, which often defeats what we know to be in our best interests.

Myths About Hypnosis

> **✤ It's A Fact!!**
> In hypnosis, the patient is not under the control of the hypnotist. Hypnosis is not something imposed on people; but something they do for themselves. A hypnotist simply serves as a facilitator to guide them.

People often fear that being hypnotized will make them lose control, surrender their will, and result in their being dominated; but a hypnotic state is not the same thing as gullibility or weakness. Many people base their assumptions about hypnotism on stage acts but fail to take into account that stage hypnotists screen their volunteers to select those who are cooperative, with possible exhibitionist tendencies, as well as responsive to hypnosis. Stage acts help create a myth about hypnosis, which discourages people from seeking legitimate hypnotherapy.

Another myth about hypnosis is that people lose consciousness and have amnesia. A small percentage of subjects who go into very deep levels of trance will fit this stereotype and have spontaneous amnesia. The majority of people remember everything that occurs in hypnosis. This is beneficial because the most of what we want to accomplish in hypnosis may be done in a medium depth trance where people tend to remember everything.

When Will Hypnosis Be Beneficial?

We believe that hypnosis will be optimally effective when the patient is highly motivated to overcome a problem and when the hypnotherapist is well trained in both hypnosis and in general considerations relating to the treatment of the particular problem. Some individuals seem to have higher native hypnotic talent and capacity that may allow them to benefit more readily from hypnosis.

It is important to keep in mind that hypnosis is like any other therapeutic modality. It is of major benefit to some patients with some problems, and it is helpful with many other patients; but it can fail just like any other clinical method. For this reason, hypnotherapists emphasize that they are not "hypnotists" but health care professionals who use hypnosis along with other tools of their profession.

Selecting A Qualified Hypnotherapist

As in choosing any health care professional, care should be exercised in selecting a hypnotherapist. Hypnosis and the use of hypnotic therapies are not regulated in most states, and hypnotherapists are, in most cases, not state licensed in hypnosis. Lay hypnotists are people who are trained in hypnosis but lack medical, psychological, dental or other professional health care training. A lay hypnotist may be certified and claim to have received 200 or more hours of training; but licensed health care professionals typically have seven to nine years of university coursework, plus additional supervised training in internship and residency programs. Their hypnosis training is in addition to their medical, psychological, dental or social work training. Careful questioning can help you avoid a lay hypnotist who may engage in fraudulent or unethical practices.

Ask if the person is licensed (not certified) in their field by the state. If they are not legitimately licensed, they probably lack the education required for licensure. Find out what their degree is in. If it is in hypnosis or hypnotherapy, rather than a state-recognized health care profession, the person is a lay hypnotist. Check for membership in the American Society of Clinical Hypnosis or the Society for Clinical and Experimental Hypnosis (which are the only nationally recognized organizations for licensed health care professionals using hypnosis) as well as membership in the American Medical Association, the American Dental Association, the American Psychological Association, etc. Contact a state or local component section of the American Society of Clinical Hypnosis to see if the person is a reputable member. If you have doubts about their qualifications, keep looking.

Uses Of Hypnosis In Medicine And Psychotherapy

Uses of hypnosis in medicine and psychotherapy include the following:

• Gastrointestinal disorders (ulcers, irritable bowel syndrome, colitis, Crohn disease)

• Dermatologic disorders (eczema, herpes, neurodermatitis, pruritus (itching), psoriasis, warts)

• Surgery/anesthesiology: In unusual circumstances, hypnosis has been used as the sole anesthetic for surgery, including the removal of the gall bladder, amputation, cesarean section, and hysterectomy. Reasons for using hypnosis as the sole anesthetic may include the following: situations where chemical anesthesia is contraindicated because of allergies or hyper-sensitivities; when organic problems increase the risk of using chemo anesthesia; and in some conditions where it is ideal for the patient to be able to respond to questions or directives from the surgeon.

• Pain (back pain, cancer pain, dental anesthesia, headaches and migraines, arthritis or rheumatism)

• Burns: Hypnosis is not only effective for the pain; but when hypnotic anesthesia and feelings of coolness are created in the first few hours after a significant burn, it appears that it also reduces inflammation and promotes healing. It is believed that a second-degree burn can often be kept from going third degree if hypnosis is used soon after the injury.

• Nausea and vomiting associated with chemotherapy and pregnancy

• Childbirth: Based upon anecdotal evidence, approximately two thirds of women have been found capable of using hypnosis as the sole analgesic for labor. This eliminates the risks that medications can pose to both the mother and child.

♣ It's A Fact!!
Uses Of Hypnosis In Dentistry

- alleviating dental anxiety
- bruxism (grinding teeth)
- gag reflex control
- adjustment to oral appliances
- anesthesia
- chronic jaw pain
- improved healing

- Hemophilia: Hemophilia patients can often be taught to use self-hypnosis to control vascular flow and keep from requiring a blood transfusion.

- Victims of abuse (incest, rape, physical abuse, cult abuse)

Other areas of application include the following: allergies, anxiety and stress management, asthma, bed wetting, depression, sports and athletic performance, smoking cessation, obesity and weight control, sleep disorders, Raynaud's disease, high blood pressure, sexual dysfunctions, concentration, test anxiety, and learning disorders.

Chapter 33

Meditation

Introduction

Meditation for health purposes is a mind-body practice in complementary and alternative medicine (CAM). There are many types of meditation, most of which originated in ancient religious and spiritual traditions. Generally, a person who is meditating uses certain techniques, such as focusing attention (for example, on a word, an object, or the breath), a specific posture, and an open attitude toward distracting thoughts and emotions. Meditation can be practiced for various reasons—for example, with intent to increase physical relaxation, mental calmness, and psychological balance; to cope with one or more diseases and conditions; and for overall wellness. This chapter provides a general introduction to meditation.

What Meditation Is

The term meditation refers to a group of techniques, most of which started in Eastern religious or spiritual traditions. These techniques have been used by many different cultures throughout the world for thousands of years. Today, many people use meditation outside of its traditional religious or cultural settings, for health and wellness purposes.

About This Chapter: Information in this chapter is from "Meditation for Health Purposes," National Center for Complementary and Alternative Medicine (NCCAM), National Institutes of Health, NCCAM Publication No. D302, January 2006.

In meditation, a person learns to focus his attention and suspend the stream of thoughts that normally occupy the mind. This practice is believed to result in a state of greater physical relaxation, mental calmness, and psychological balance. Practicing meditation can change how a person relates to the flow of emotions and thoughts in the mind.

Most types of meditation have four elements in common:

- **A quiet location.** Many meditators prefer a quiet place with as few distractions as possible. This can be particularly helpful for beginners. People who have been practicing meditation for a longer period of time sometimes develop the ability to meditate in public places, like waiting rooms or buses.

- **A specific, comfortable posture.** Depending on the type being practiced, meditation can be done while sitting, lying down, standing, walking, or in other positions.

- **A focus of attention.** Focusing one's attention is usually a part of meditation. For example, the meditator may focus on a mantra (a specially chosen word or set of words), an object, or the breath.

- **An open attitude.** Having an open attitude during meditation means letting distractions come and go naturally without stopping to think about them. When distracting or wandering thoughts occur, they are not suppressed; instead, the meditator gently brings attention back to the focus. In some types of meditation, the meditator learns to observe the rising and falling of thoughts and emotions as they spontaneously occur.

Meditation is practiced both on its own and as a component of some other therapies, such as yoga, tai chi, and qigong. This chapter focuses on meditation practiced on its own.

Meditation For Health Purposes

Meditation, used as CAM, is a type of mind-body medicine (one of the four domains, or areas of knowledge, in CAM). Generally, mind-body medicine focuses on the following:

- The interactions among the brain, the rest of the body, the mind, and behavior

- The ways in which emotional, mental, social, spiritual, and behavioral factors can directly affect health

People use meditation for various health problems, such as these:

- Anxiety

- Pain

- Depression

- Mood and self-esteem problems

- Stress

- Insomnia

- Physical or emotional symptoms that may be associated with chronic illnesses and their treatment, such as the following:

  - Cardiovascular (heart) disease

  - HIV/AIDS

  - Cancer

Meditation is also used for overall wellness.

A large national survey on Americans' use of CAM, released in 2004, found that nearly 8 percent of the participants had used meditation specifically for health reasons during the year before the survey.

Examples Of Meditation

Mindfulness meditation and the transcendental meditation technique (also known as TM) are two common approaches to meditation. They are also two types of meditation being studied in NCCAM-sponsored research projects.

Mindfulness meditation originated in Buddhism. It is based on the concept of being mindful, or having an increased awareness and total acceptance of the present. While meditating, the meditator is taught to bring all her attention to the sensation of the flow of the breath in and out of the body. The intent might be described as focusing attention on what is being

♣ It's A Fact!!
Meditation May Reduce Heart Disease Risk

Black adolescents with high normal blood pressure who practice transcendental meditation improve the ability of their blood vessels to relax and may reduce their risk of becoming adults with cardiovascular disease, researchers say.

After eight months of meditation, these adolescents experienced a 21 percent increase in the ability of their blood vessels to dilate compared to a 4 percent decrease experienced by their non-meditating peers, says Dr. Vernon A. Barnes, physiologist at the Medical College of Georgia's (MCG) Georgia Prevention Institute and lead investigator on the study.

"Our blood vessels are not rigid pipes," says Dr. Barnes. "They need to dilate and constrict, according to the needs of the body. If this improvement in the ability to dilate can be replicated in other at-risk groups and cardiovascular disease patients, this could have important implications for inclusion of meditation programs to prevent and treat cardiovascular disease and its clinical consequences.

"We know this type of change is achievable with lipid lowering drugs, but it's remarkable that a meditation program can produce such a change," the researcher says.

In the April 2004 issue of the *American Journal of Hypertension*, Dr. Barnes and his colleagues reported that 15 minutes of twice-daily transcendental meditation steadily lowered the blood pressure of 156 black, inner-city adolescents and their pressures tended to stay lower.

This new study focused on 111 of those adolescents, 57 who meditated and 54 controls.

MCG researchers found among the meditators an increased ability of the blood vessel lining, called the endothelium, to relax. "Dysfunction in the ability of the endothelium to dilate is an early event in heart disease, a process that starts at a young age," says Dr. Barnes.

At four months and again at eight months, researchers used echocardiography to measure the diameter of the right brachial artery, the main artery that feeds the arm, before and after a blood pressure cuff was inflated for two minutes.

They found essentially no difference in the ability of that vessel to relax after stress in either group at four months. But by eight months, EDAD, or endothelial-dependent arterial dilation, was significantly improved in the meditators, says Dr. Barnes, noting that as with all lifestyle changes, the full benefits of meditating may take a while.

"Change can't be expected overnight," he says. "Meditation and other positive lifestyle habits, such as exercising and eating right, have to become part of your life, like brushing your teeth." Long-term studies are needed to determine the long-term impact of meditation on the risk of heart disease, he says.

Doctors already know that smoking, high blood pressure and cholesterol, and cardiovascular disease are all associated with decreased EDAD. "With the high prevalence of heart disease we have in our country today, this is something that should be considered," he says of meditation, which is inexpensive and has no side effects.

The obesity epidemic in the United States, he says, likely is the primary contributor to the increasing blood pressure rates in children. But obesity appears to be part of an unhealthy cycle where the stresses of everyday life, such as poverty and not feeling safe at home, contribute to bad habits such as overeating and/or eating high-fat comfort foods and not exercising. Stress also may impair sleep, preventing the body, and blood pressure, from resting and recovering.

It appears that meditating—allowing the mind to settle to minimal activity for 15 minutes twice daily—may help the meditator and his blood vessels relax in the hectic world around him.

Dr. Frank Treiber, director of MCG's Georgia Prevention Institute, and Dr. Surender Malhotra, cardiology fellow at MCG, are co-authors on the study which is highlighted as one of 10 abstract submissions to the conference viewed as having the highest potential to change clinical practice from the perspective of screening, diagnosis or treatment.

The National Heart, Lung and Blood Institute funded the research.

Source: "Meditation may reduce heart disease risk," March 2, 2005. Reprinted with permission from the Medical College of Georgia.

experienced, without reacting to or judging that experience. This is seen as helping the meditator learn to experience thoughts and emotions in normal daily life with greater balance and acceptance.

TM originated in the Vedic tradition in India. It is a type of meditation that uses a mantra (a word, sound, or phrase repeated silently) to prevent distracting thoughts from entering the mind. The intent of TM might be described as allowing the mind to settle into a quieter state and the body into a state of deep rest. This is seen as ultimately leading to a state of relaxed alertness.

Looking At How Meditation May Work

Practicing meditation has been shown to induce some changes in the body, such as changes in the body's "fight or flight" response. The system responsible for this response is the autonomic nervous system (sometimes called the involuntary nervous system). It regulates many organs and muscles, including functions such as the heartbeat, sweating, breathing, and digestion, and does so automatically.

The autonomic nervous system is divided into two parts, which are as follows:

- The **sympathetic nervous system** helps mobilize the body for action. When a person is under stress, it produces the fight-or-flight response: the heart rate and breathing rate go up, for example, the blood vessels narrow (restricting the flow of blood), and muscles tighten.

- The **parasympathetic nervous system** creates what some call the "rest and digest" response. This system's responses oppose those of the sympathetic nervous system. For example, it causes the heart rate and breathing rate to slow down, the blood vessels to dilate (improving blood flow), and activity to increase in many parts of the digestive tract.

While scientists are studying whether meditation may afford meaningful health benefits, they are also looking at how it may do so. One way some types of meditation might work is by reducing activity in the sympathetic nervous system and increasing activity in the parasympathetic nervous system.

Scientific research is using sophisticated tools to learn more about what goes on in the brain and the rest of the body during meditation, and diseases or conditions for which meditation might be useful. There is still much to learn in these areas. One avenue of research is looking at whether meditation is associated with significant changes in brain function. A number of researchers believe that these changes account for many of meditation's effects.

Side Effects And Risks

Meditation is generally safe. There have been a small number of reports that intensive meditation could cause or worsen symptoms in people who have certain psychiatric problems, but this question has not been fully researched. Individuals who are aware of an underlying psychiatric disorder and want to start meditation should speak with a mental health professional before doing so.

Any person who is interested in using meditation, as CAM, should consider the following:

- Meditation should never delay the time it takes you to see your health care provider about having a medical problem diagnosed or treated, and it should not be used as the only treatment without first consulting your provider.

- It is important to discuss any CAM therapies you are considering or using (including meditation) with your provider for a complete treatment plan and your safety.

- If you are interested in learning meditation, ask about the training and experience of the instructor.

- Find out whether there have been any research studies published on meditation for the health condition you are interested in.

NCCAM-Supported Research

Some recent studies supported by NCCAM have been investigating the following:

- The potential effectiveness of the transcendental meditation technique to prevent and treat heart disease

- Mindfulness-based stress reduction to relieve symptoms of rheuma-toid arthritis and, in a different study, chronic lower back pain

- What happens to the brain's activity and structures during Buddhist insight meditation (which includes mindfulness) in a study that uses a brain scan called fMRI (functional magnetic resonance imaging)

- The long-term impact of meditation on basic emotional and cognitive functions and on mechanisms in the brain that are involved in these functions

Chapter 34

Prayer And Spirituality

People have used prayer and other spiritual practices for their own and others' health concerns for thousands of years. Scientific investigation of these practices has begun quite recently, however, to better understand whether they work; if so, how; and for what diseases/conditions and populations. The National Center for Complementary and Alternative Medicine (NCCAM) is supporting research in this arena.

Many Americans are using prayer and other spiritual practices. This was confirmed by findings from the largest and most comprehensive survey to date on Americans' use of complementary and alternative medicine. This survey of more than 31,000 adults, released in May 2004 by the National Center for Health Statistics and NCCAM, found that 36 percent had used complementary and alternative medicine (CAM), when prayer was not included in the definition of CAM; when prayer was included in the definition of CAM, 62 percent had used CAM (all figures refer to use in the preceding 12 months). Among the respondents the following was found:

- 45 percent had used prayer for health reasons.

- 43 percent had prayed for their own health.

About This Chapter: Information in this chapter is excerpted from "Prayer and Spirituality in Health: Ancient Practices, Modern Science," *CAM at the NIH*, Volume XII, Number 1, Winter 2005, National Center for Complementary and Alternative Medicine (NCCAM), National Institutes of Health.

- Almost 25 percent had had others pray for them.

- Almost 10 percent had participated in a prayer group for their health.

Prayer was the therapy most commonly used among the entire CAM therapies included in the survey. The report also addressed the use of other CAM approaches that can have a spiritual component, including meditation, yoga, tai chi, qigong, and Reiki.

Catherine Stoney, Ph.D., a Program Officer in NCCAM's Division of Extramural Research and Training, oversees many grants in NCCAM's mind-body portfolio. She noted: "There is already some preliminary evidence for a connection between prayer and related practices and health outcomes. For example, we've seen some evidence that religious affiliation and religious practices are associated with health and mortality—in other words, with better health and longer life. Such connections may involve immune function, cardiovascular function, and/or other physiological changes." However, she added, this is by no means proven. "For some individuals, religious practices are an effective way of coping with stress, and the beneficial health effects may come about by reducing stress. For others, religious practices may not result in reduced stress or be associated with health benefits. It can be challenging to separate out these effects because people have different ideas regarding the meaning of various practices. For this reason, we are particularly interested in understanding the impact of personal, positive meaning on health."

♣ It's A Fact!!

Within complementary and alternative medicine (CAM), prayer is defined by the National Center for Complementary and Alternative Medicine (NCCAM) as an active process of appealing to a higher spiritual power, specifically for health reasons; it includes individual or group prayer on behalf of oneself or others. Spirituality is broader; it is defined by NCCAM as an individual's sense of purpose and meaning to life, beyond material values. Spirituality may be practiced in many ways, including through religion.

Other challenges in this very new field of research include the following:

- The fact that different researchers have defined prayer, spirituality, and related concepts in different ways

- A relative lack of standardized questionnaires (compared with many other fields of medicine)

Snapshots Of NCCAM Research

NCCAM is funding several studies of prayer and other explicitly spiritual practices. Goals range from improving quality of life, to looking at the impact of these practices on the immune system and on serious chronic health conditions, to assisting people through the end of life.

Spirituality In The Context Of Chronic Illness

Joel Tsevat, M.D., Director of Outcomes Research in the Department of Internal Medicine at the University of Cincinnati, is completing a study of the will to live in patients with HIV/AIDS. His team is using several standardized tools that measure different aspects of spirituality, such as a sense of meaning and peace and faith, religious coping measures, and involvement in organized and non-organized religious activity. They are also looking at measures of health status, health concerns, depression, self-esteem, and social support. The study involves interviews with 350 individuals with HIV/AIDS in Cincinnati and Washington, D.C.

Dr. Tsevat became interested in studying spirituality during earlier research with patients with HIV/AIDS. "Patients were telling us that they had discovered new meaning and purpose in their lives since being diagnosed with HIV," Dr. Tsevat said. "The spirituality theme emerged when we asked patients whether they would choose their health as it is or take a gamble between death and perfect health." People who were spiritual tended to be happier with their current health status and less likely to take the described risk.

"We tend to focus just on what medical professionals can address—physical functioning and mental health," said Dr. Tsevat. "In the scheme of things, I think spiritual well-being is also an important component of someone's quality of life."

Spirituality, Immunity, And Emotional Well-Being

Several NCCAM-supported researchers in New York City are exploring the impact of spirituality on the immune system and its role in emotional well-being among cancer patients.

Barry Rosenfeld, Ph.D., and graduate student Colleen McClain, M.A., of Fordham University, and William Breitbart, M.D., of Memorial Sloan-Kettering Cancer Center, published results in 2003 of an NCCAM-funded study on the effect of spiritual well-being on end-of-life despair in terminally ill cancer patients. They concluded that spiritual well-being offers some protection—a buffer effect—against end-of-life despair in patients for whom death is imminent. These researchers are now studying spirituality-based interventions to establish methods that can help engender a sense of peace and meaning.

"When people despair, they feel nothing they've done has had any meaning. We help them remember things they've forgotten during the throes of their illness so they can realistically place themselves in the world," Dr. Rosenfeld said. The approach is spiritually based, he said, but "we have tried to not have it linked to any particular religious framework, keeping it open to as many individuals who are interested."

To determine whether immune function is a link between spirituality and emotional well-being, the three researchers are also now collaborating, under another NCCAM grant, to measure spirituality and interleukin-6 (IL-6) levels in the blood among terminally ill cancer patients. "There is a small, but growing, body of literature linking immune function to mood, and IL-6 is the immune marker most highly correlated with mood states," Dr. Rosenfeld said. IL-6 is a protein that acts on other cells to regulate immune system function. It is one of several markers of inflammation, an important process in a variety of diseases like heart disease, diabetes, and stroke, and is associated with increased stress and depression.

Chapter 35

Qigong

Qigong is an ancient Chinese health care system that integrates physical postures, breathing techniques, and focused intention.

The word qigong (chi kung) is made up of two Chinese words. Qi is pronounced "chee" and is usually translated to mean the life force or vital-energy that flows through all things in the universe.

The second word, gong, pronounced "gung", means accomplishment, or skill that is cultivated through steady practice. Together, qigong (chi kung) means cultivating energy. It is a system practiced for health maintenance, healing, and increasing vitality.

Qigong practices can be classified as martial, medical, or spiritual. All styles have three things in common. They all involve a posture, (whether moving or stationary), breathing techniques, and mental focus. Some practices increase the qi; others circulate it, use it to cleanse and heal the body, store it, or emit qi to help heal others. Practices vary from the soft internal styles such as tai chi to the external, vigorous styles such as kung fu. However, the slow gentle movements of most qigong forms can be easily adapted, even for the physically challenged and can be practiced by all age groups.

About This Chapter: Information in this chapter is from "What is Qigong?" © 2006 National Qigong Association. All rights reserved. Reprinted with permission.

Like any other system of health care, qigong is not a panacea, but it is certainly a highly effective health care practice. Many health care professionals recommend qigong as an important form of alternative complementary medicine.

✣ **It's A Fact!!**
Qigong is an integration of physical postures, breathing techniques, and focused intentions.

Qigong creates an awareness of and influences dimensions of our being that are not part of traditional exercise programs. Most exercises do not involve the meridian system used in acupuncture nor do they emphasize the importance of adding mind intent and breathing techniques to physical movements. When these dimensions are added, the benefits of exercise increase exponentially.

The gentle, rhythmic movements of qigong reduce stress, build stamina, increase vitality, and enhance the immune system. It has also been found to improve cardiovascular, respiratory, circulatory, lymphatic, and digestive functions.

Those who maintain a consistent practice of qigong find that it helps one regain a youthful vitality, maintain health even into old age, and helps speed recovery from illness. Western scientific research confirms that qigong reduces hypertension and the incidence of falling in the aged population. One of the more important long-term effects is that qigong re-establishes the body/mind/soul connection.

People do qigong to maintain health, heal their bodies, calm their minds, and reconnect with their spirit.

When these three aspects of our being are integrated, it encourages a positive outlook on life and helps eliminate harmful attitudes and behaviors. It also creates a balanced life style, which brings greater harmony, stability, and enjoyment.

There are a wide variety of qigong practices. They vary from the simple, internal forms to the more complex and challenging external styles. They can interest and benefit everyone, from the most physically challenged to the super athlete. There are qigong classes for children, senior citizens, and every age group in between. Since qigong can be practiced anywhere or at any time, there is no need to buy special clothing or to join a health club.

Qigong's great appeal is that everyone can benefit, regardless of ability, age, belief system, or life circumstances.

Anyone can enrich their lives by adding qigong to their daily routine—children learning to channel their energy and develop increased concentration; office workers learning qigong to reduce stress; seniors participating in gentle movements to enhance balance and their quality of life; caregivers embracing a practice to develop their ability to help others; prisons instituting qigong programs to restore balance in inmates lives; midwives using qigong techniques to ease child birth.

Chapter 36

Tai Chi

What is tai chi?

Tai chi, pronounced "tie chee," is a gentle exercise program that is a part of traditional Chinese medicine. Derived from the martial arts, tai chi is composed of slow, deliberate movements, meditation, and deep breathing, which enhance physical health and emotional well-being.

As are many practices from the East, tai chi is based on spiritual and philosophical ideas that advocate a need for balance in the body, mind, and spirit. Central to tai chi is the idea that qi (pronounced "chee"), or life energy, flows throughout the body. Qi must be able to move freely for good health. The principle of yin/yang is important, too. Yin and yang are opposite and complementary forces in the universe, such as light and dark. Tai chi is meant to harmonize these pairs of opposites. Finally, tai chi imitates motion found in nature, such as the movements of animals, thereby uniting human beings with the natural world.

What is the history of tai chi?

Zhang Sanfeng, a martial artist who lived in China in the late 16th century, created the practice of tai chi. According to legend, Sanfeng had a dream

about a snake and a crane engaged in battle. Their graceful movements inspired his non-combative style of martial arts. This ancient form of movement
has been practiced in China for centuries and is still a daily routine for tens of
thousands of people there, especially the elderly. It was first introduced to the
United States in the early 1970s and has since grown in popularity.

How does tai chi work?

There are various perspectives on how tai chi works. Eastern philosophy
holds that tai chi unblocks the flow of qi. When qi flows properly, the body,
mind, and spirit are in balance and health is maintained. Others believe that
tai chi works in the same way as other mind/body therapies, and there is ample
evidence that paying attention to the connection between the mind and the
body can relieve stress, combat disease, and enhance physical well-being.

Tai chi has three major components. They are the following:

- **Movement:** All the major muscle groups and joints are needed for the
  slow, gentle movements in tai chi. Tai chi improves balance, agility,
  strength, flexibility, stamina, muscle tone, and coordination. This low-
  impact, weight-bearing exercise strengthens bones and can slow bone
  loss, thus preventing the development of osteoporosis.

- **Meditation:** Research shows that meditation soothes the mind, enhances concentration, reduces anxiety, and lowers blood pressure and
  heart rate.

- **Deep breathing:** Exhaling stale air and toxins from the lungs while
  inhaling a plenitude of fresh air increases lung capacity, stretches
  the muscles involved in breathing, and releases tension. It also enhances blood circulation to the brain, which boosts mental alertness.
  At the same time, the entire body is supplied with fresh oxygen and
  nutrients.

What does a tai chi session entail?

Tai chi sessions are usually group classes that last about an hour. Each
session begins with a warm-up exercise. Then the instructor guides the class
through a series of 20 to 100 tai chi movements that together comprise a

"form." A form can take up to 20 minutes to complete. Each form has a nature-based name that describes its overall action—such as "wave hands like clouds" or "grasp the bird's tail." At the same time, students are asked to focus on the point just below their navels, believed to be the center from which qi flows. The teacher encourages the class to perform all movements in a slow, meditative manner and to focus on deep breathing. At the end of the class, there is usually a wind-down exercise, relaxation, and meditation.

How many sessions will I need?

Classes are usually taught on a weekly basis. Many practitioners recommend practicing tai chi for about 15 to 20 minutes twice daily at home, since regular practice is essential for mastering the forms and achieving lasting results. Before beginning a tai chi program, you should check with your doctor and discuss your health needs with the tai chi instructor. Exercises can be modified depending on your mobility, history of injuries, chronic pain, joint swelling (if present), and medication that may affect balance.

♣ It's A Fact!!
Tai chi improves overall fitness, coordination, and agility. People who practice tai chi on a regular basis tend to have good posture, flexibility, and range of motion, are more mentally alert, and sleep more soundly at night.

What conditions respond well to tai chi?

Tai chi is both a preventive and a complementary therapy for a wide range of conditions. Specifically, it is beneficial for chronic pain, gout, heart disease, high blood pressure, arthritis, osteoporosis, headaches, and sleep disorders. Tai chi is also beneficial for the immune system and the central nervous system, which makes it especially good for people with a chronic illness, anxiety, depression, or any stress-related conditions. The deep breathing of tai chi regulates the respiratory system, helping to treat respiratory ailments such as asthma, bronchitis, and emphysema. It also stimulates the abdomen, which aids digestion and helps relieve constipation and gastrointestinal conditions. Many studies indicate that elderly people who practice tai chi are much less prone to falls, a serious health risk to people in that age group.

Are there conditions that should not be treated with tai chi?

Tai chi is safe for everyone, regardless of age or athletic ability, and can be modified for most health problems. People with limited mobility—even those in wheelchairs—can learn and successfully use tai chi; however, it is not meant to replace medical care for a serious condition. Talk to your doctor and your instructor about any health problems or recent injuries you may have.

Is there anything I should look out for?

Tai chi exercises muscles in areas of your body that may have been neglected for a while. Therefore, you may feel sore in the beginning. It takes time to develop the posture, flexibility, and agility needed for tai chi, so don't get discouraged. As with any exercise program, safety is affected by proper stretching and warm-up exercises, as well as correct alignment. If you experience dizziness, shortness of breath, headaches, or severe pain, stop practicing and talk to your instructor right away, and consult your doctor.

How can I find a qualified tai chi practitioner?

For information on how to find a tai chi class in your area, contact your local health club or YMCA. Ask to sit in on a class before signing up, so that you can observe the instructor and the atmosphere of the class.

Chapter 37

Yoga

What is yoga?

Yoga, derived from the Sanskrit word meaning "union," is a spiritual practice that uses the body, breath, and mind to energize and balance the whole person. This mind-body therapy involves physical postures, breathing exercises, and meditation to improve overall well being. Yoga began nearly 6,000 years ago in India as part of the Hindu healing science known as Ayurveda. Today, approximately six million Americans practice yoga regularly.

What is the history of yoga?

While the practice of yoga started nearly 6,000 years ago, the earliest written records documenting yoga as a health practice are recorded in The Vedas, texts from India dating back at least three thousand years. There have been other ancient texts documenting the philosophy and teachings of yoga; however, yoga did not emerge as a fully developed practice until 500 B.C. In its traditional form, yoga is considered a complete lifestyle that provides a path to spiritual enlightenment.

The practice of yoga came to the United States in the 1890s as a result of the teachings of a guru named Swami Vivekananda. It gained popularity in the 1960s because of a rising interest in, and cultural acceptance of, alternative

About This Chapter: Information in this chapter is from "Yoga." © 2006 A.D.A.M., Inc. Reprinted with permission.

modalities and mind-body therapies. Today, yoga is often practiced as an exercise form separated from its traditional spiritual roots. In this form, yoga exercise is taught at local YMCAs, health clubs, and yoga centers, and is often part of disease prevention and management programs in hospitals, such as stress-reduction courses for people with high blood pressure and heart disease.

Are there different types of yoga?

As the different connections between the mind and body were explored, various branches of yoga developed. These include in the following:

- **Astanga or Power Yoga:** Modern day variations of yoga developed for people who prefer a physically demanding workout.

- **Bhakti Yoga:** The goal of this form of yoga is to take all of the love in one's heart and direct it to God. By worshiping God, the person who practices regularly becomes filled with respect for all life and is encouraged to be sacrificial and to treat others generously.

- **Bikram Yoga:** A series of 26 asanas (postures) practiced in a room that is 105 degrees in order to warm and stretch the muscles, ligaments, and tendons and to detoxify the body through sweat.

- **Hatha Yoga:** The most commonly practiced form of yoga in the United States today. Emphasis is placed on physical postures or exercises, known as asanas, with the goal of balancing the opposites in one's life. During Hatha yoga sessions, flexing is followed by extension, a rounded back is followed by an arched back, and physical exercises are followed by mental meditations.

- **Iyangar Yoga:** Emphasizes great attention to detail and precise alignment. This often requires the use of props such as blocks and belts while performing postures.

- **Jnana Yoga:** Emphasizes deep contemplation. Practitioners seek Jnana, or "wisdom," through meditation. The goal of this form of yoga is to be one with God.

> **♣ It's A Fact!!**
> The branches of yoga incorporate three major techniques:
> - Breathing
> - Exercise (asana or postures)
> - Meditation

- **Karma Yoga:** Based on the philosophy that "yesterday's actions determine today's circumstances." Practitioners of Karma yoga make a conscious decision to perform selfless acts of kindness. By making today's actions positive, they hope they can improve tomorrow's circumstances for both themselves as well as others.

- **Raja Yoga:** Known in India as "the royal (raj) road to reintegration." The goal of this type of yoga is to blend the four layers of self: the body, the individual consciousness, the individual sub-consciousness, and the universal and infinite consciousness. Raja yoga, being most concerned with the mind and spirit, places its emphasis on meditation.

- **Tantra Yoga:** Like Hatha yoga, practitioners of Tantra yoga seek to balance the opposites in their lives. They also try to break free of the "six enemies" (physical longing, anger, greed, vanity, obsession, jealousy) and the "eight fetters" (hatred, apprehension, fear, shyness, hypocrisy, pride of ancestry, vanity of culture, egotism) by using discipline, training, and rituals.

How does yoga work?

Scientists don't know exactly how yoga produces its healthful effects. Some say it works like other mind-body therapies to reduce stress, and others believe that yoga promotes the release of endorphins (natural painkillers and mood elevators) from the brain.

All of the branches of yoga previously mentioned incorporate three major techniques: breathing, exercise (asana or postures), and meditation. These three techniques have been shown to improve health in the following ways:

- **Breathing lessons:** In yoga, breath work is known as pranayama. Pranayama increases blood circulation and reduces oxygen consumption, which brings more oxygen to the brain, and improves the efficiency of oxygen use in the body. Also, as lung tissue becomes more elastic and the surrounding muscle more flexible, the practice of pranayama can also increase lung capacity. Getting ample air into our lungs helps us to feel alert and focused.

- **Asanas (postures):** Provide a gentle workout that enhances strength, flexibility, and balance. Some asanas are designed to massage the internal organs, improve circulation, hormone function, digestion, and other body processes.

- **Meditation:** Stills the mind and induces both physical and emotional relaxation. In so doing, it reduces blood pressure, chronic pain, anxiety, and cholesterol levels.

What does a yoga session entail?

Although most people learn yoga by taking a group class with an experienced instructor, one-to-one sessions with certain practitioners are available. Such private, or semi-private, sessions tend to be quite costly. Classes usually last from 45 to 90 minutes and begin with warm-up exercises, proceed to a guided series of yoga postures designed to stretch and tone all areas of the body, and generally end with deep relaxation and/or meditation. Throughout the class, the teacher instructs you on breath control and proper body alignment.

How many sessions will I need?

Classes are generally taken once a week (or more, if desired). Your instructor will likely encourage you to practice at home to get the most from yoga.

What is yoga good for?

Yoga improves fitness, lowers blood pressure, promotes relaxation and self-confidence, and reduces stress and anxiety. People who practice yoga tend to have good coordination, posture, flexibility, range of motion, concentration, sleep habits, and digestion.

Studies show that yoga may promote heart health in both the young and old. An analysis of scientific studies found that yoga might help manage heart disease by doing the following:

- Decreasing high blood pressure

- Lowering cholesterol levels

- Increasing resistance to stress

✤ It's A Fact!!

Yoga is a complementary therapy that has been used with conventional therapies to help treat a wide range of health problems; but it is not, in and of itself, an effective cure for any particular disease.

• Reducing the frequency and severity of chest pain (if yoga is combined with a healthy diet)

More research suggests that yoga may help people with asthma. For example, people who practice yoga postures and breathing exercises tend to breathe easier and more efficiently. One study also found that people with asthma used their inhalers less often when they were practicing yoga.

Yoga postures aimed at stretching and strengthening the joints in the upper body can improve grip strength and diminish pain among people with carpal tunnel syndrome. Yoga may also be effective for managing pain and enhancing range of motion in people with osteoarthritis.

Other conditions that seem to be responsive to yoga include the following:

• Back pain

• Anxiety

• Irritability

• Feelings of sadness or depression

• Ability to help prevent type 2 diabetes

• Various conditions before, during, and after pregnancy

Is there anything I should look out for?

Some people may experience stiffness as their bodies adapt to different postures. Plus, as with any physical activity, yoga may lead to an injury if not practiced properly. This is why practicing yoga under the guidance of a trained professional is important. Avoid yoga if you've had a recent back injury, and be sure to check with your doctor before trying yoga if you have high blood pressure, heart disease, or arthritis, as you would any physical activity. In addition, if you have any of these conditions, choose one of the gentler forms of yoga discussed earlier. Some postures are not recommended during pregnancy, but special classes are available for pregnant women. Some postures should not be practiced during menstruation. Be sure to contact your doctor if any exercises cause headaches, muscle cramps, dizziness, or severe pain in your back, legs, or joints.

Part Six

Biologically Based Practices And Energy Medicine

Chapter 38

Apitherapy

What is apitherapy?

As a technique, it is the medical use of the products of the honeybee hive, often used with essential oils.

As a philosophy, it is a form of harmony between the individual and the environment.

As a medical principle, it is primarily the cultivation of health and its re-establishment when sickness interferes.

What products are used in apitherapy?

They are honey, pollen, propolis, royal jelly, and bee venom. These products can be used individually. More frequently, several of those are used together. Essential oils, already present in honey and propolis, are often used in conjunction with the products of the hive.

What kinds of conditions are treated with apitherapy?

Currently the most popular and well-known uses of honeybee venom in the United States are for people suffering from multiple sclerosis (MS) and many forms of arthritis. Now, the only condition that has actual scientific data supporting the use of apitherapy for treatment is post-herpetic neuralgia. There were several articles written in the first half of the 1900s about using bee venom in the treatment of osteoarthritis and rheumatoid arthritis, and there is some ongoing research now looking at it's effect in multiple sclerosis. Anecdotal reports suggest that it might have some usefulness in the treatment of infectious, autoimmune, cardiovascular, pulmonary, gastrointestinal, neuropathic pain, and other chronic pain conditions.

How are MS and arthritis treated?

Bee venom, in synergy with other bee products, is the major therapeutic agent. Live bee stings or a commercially available venom extract, which doctors can inject, are used in conjunction with one or more of the products of the beehive mentioned previously.

Where can I find someone who can help me with apitherapy?

The American Apitherapy Society (AAS) has information in its database of practitioners and of people ready to give information and assistance. This information is available to society members.

Who practices apitherapy?

Practitioners include physicians, nurses, acupuncturists, naturopaths, as well as interested laypersons including bee keepers, who can provide persons with bees who want bee venom therapy and instruct them how to treat themselves.

✎ What's It Mean?

Essential Oils: Oils that come from plants, fruits, and flowers. [1]

Propolis: A resinous product collected from beehives. [2]

Royal Jelly: Food secreted by worker bees and placed in queen cells for larval food. [3]

Source: [1] Editor. [2] "Whole Medical Systems: An Overview," National Center for Complimentary and Alternative Medicine, NCCAM Publication No. D236, October 2004. [3] "Honey: Background for 1995 Farm Legislation," U.S. Department of Agriculture, Economic Research Service.

Is apitherapy covered by insurance?

No, however, many AAS member practitioners do not charge for the procedure, but some do charge for their time. A donation to AAS is appreciated to support the dissemination of information about apitherapy. The amount of the donation can vary and can be discussed with the practitioner. Joining the AAS is another way to support the organization, and you get an informative and entertaining newsletter quarterly as part of the membership.

Is apitherapy a recognized therapy in the United States?

No official body in the United States has sanctioned apitherapy as a recognized treatment modality. The Food and Drug Administration, for desensitization purposes only, has approved bee venom.

What about bee sting allergy? I had a bee sting me once and swelled up a lot. I was told I am allergic. Can I still get bee venom therapy?

Contrary to popular belief, allergy to honeybee sting is relatively rare. About seven in a thousand persons are allergic. Of this proportion, only a small percentage risks anaphylactic shock. Nevertheless, bee venom treatment is always to be preceded by a test of sensitivity. A sensitive person can be de-sensitized to bee venom, thus allowing apitherapy to proceed. AAS recommends that anyone who uses or administers bee venom have readily available an Epinephrine kit to be used in case of anaphylactic response and know how to use it. Erroneously, many people consider swelling after a sting to be an allergic reaction. Swelling is a normal response of the body as are localized redness, swelling, and itching.

Chapter 39

Chelation Therapy

For more than 30 years, people with fatty buildups of plaque in their arteries (atherosclerosis) may have heard about a "miracle cure" called chelation (pronounced "ke-LA' shun") therapy. But you may not know that the American Heart Association and other medical and scientific groups have spoken out against this treatment.

This chapter answers the most frequently asked questions about chelation therapy.

What is atherosclerosis?

Atherosclerosis is also called "hardening of the arteries." It occurs when the inner walls of the arteries become lined with deposits of fat, cholesterol, and other substances, including calcium. This fatty buildup usually starts early in life and gradually gets worse over many years. That is why middle-aged and older people are more likely to have the disease.

As plaque builds up, the arteries become hard and constricted. They lose their ability to expand and contract as blood flows through them and they

About This Chapter: Information in this chapter is from "Questions and Answers About Chelation Therapy." Reproduced with permission from http://www.americanheart.org. © 2005 American Heart Association.

get narrower. These changes make it harder for blood to flow through them, so the heart must work harder to pump blood throughout the body.

If this plaque ruptures or a blood clot blocks a narrowed artery, a heart attack, stroke, or other serious medical problem can result. A heart attack happens when an artery bringing blood to the heart muscle is blocked. A stroke occurs when an artery to the brain is blocked.

What is chelation therapy?

Chelation therapy is administering a man-made amino acid called EDTA into the veins. (EDTA is an abbreviation for ethylenediamine tetraacetic acid. It is marketed under several names, including Edetate, Disodium, Endrate, and Sodium Versenate.) EDTA is most often used in cases of heavy metal poisoning (lead or mercury). That is because it can latch onto or bind these metals, creating a compound that can be excreted in the urine.

Besides binding heavy metals, EDTA also "chelates" (naturally seeks out and binds) calcium, one of the components of atherosclerotic plaque. In the early 1960s, this led to speculation that EDTA could remove calcium deposits from buildups in arteries. The idea was that once the calcium was removed by regular treatments of EDTA, the remaining elements in the plaque would break up and the plaque would clear away. The narrowed arteries would be restored to their former state.

Based upon this thinking, chelation therapy has been proposed to treat existing atherosclerosis and to prevent it from forming.

After carefully reviewing all the available scientific literature on this subject, the American Heart Association has concluded that the benefits claimed for this form of therapy are not scientifically proven. That is why the American Heart Association does not recommend this type of treatment.

How long does chelation therapy last, and how much does it cost?

A single chelation treatment usually lasts from two to four hours and costs between $50 and $100. In the first month, patients usually receive from five to 30 treatments (with 30 being most common). Patients often are advised to continue preventive treatment once a month.

Patients must pay for this treatment themselves. EDTA is not a medically accepted procedure for atherosclerosis, so insurance companies and Medicare will not reimburse for it.

Is there any proof that chelation therapy works?

Supporters of chelation therapy rely on the testimonies of people who have had it done. Many people claim that their lives were saved and their health improved because of chelation therapy.

But these are not the only claims. Supporters also claim that chelation therapy significantly improves blood flow through previously narrowed blood vessels in some patients. Another claim is that chelation therapy has restored lost bodily function and reduced pain in some cases.

The American Heart Association cannot say why some people feel better after having chelation therapy. And the American Heart Association does not deny that some people actually may feel better after treatment. So what is the problem?

The problem is, the American Heart Association questions whether these patients feel better because of chelation therapy. It is possible they feel better because of something else.

For example, chelation therapists usually require their patients to make lifestyle changes. This can include quitting smoking, losing weight, eating more fruits and vegetables, avoiding foods high in saturated fats, and exercising regularly. These are healthy changes for anyone to make, and patients make them at the same time that they are undergoing chelation therapy. That is what clouds the issue. Research has shown that these lifestyle changes improve patients' quality of life and sense of well-being. In fact, the American Heart Association has advocated these lifestyle changes for many years.

The American Heart Association believes that these lifestyle changes are probably why the condition of some patients improves. The American Heart Association believes they do not feel better because of chelation therapy with EDTA, but because of better, healthier habits that they adopt.

Patients also may feel better for psychological reasons. Sometimes a sick person's symptoms disappear for no apparent reason, due
to a placebo effect. This could be why some
patients report that they feel better after
they have spent $3,000 to $5,000 for chelation therapy.

Can chelation therapy be dangerous?

EDTA is not totally safe as a drug. There is
a real danger of kidney failure (renal tubular ne-
crosis). EDTA can also cause bone marrow depression,
shock, low blood pressure (hypotension), convulsions, disturbances of regular
heart rhythm (cardiac arrhythmias), allergic-type reactions, and respiratory
arrest.

> ♣ **It's A Fact!!**
> A number of deaths in
> the United States have been
> linked with chelation therapy.
> Also, some people are on di-
> alysis because of kidney fail-
> ure caused, at least in part,
> by chelation therapy.

The American Heart Association is concerned that some people who rely
on this therapy may delay undergoing proven therapies like drugs or surgery
until it is too late. This is the added danger of relying on an unproven "miracle
cure."

Clearly, people who choose chelation therapy are risking more than money.

Chapter 40

Crystal And Gemstone Therapy

Crystal therapy is the use of crystals and gemstones to promote healing within the human body. The therapy is not limited to physical ailments, but advocates believe that these stones have a place in treating mental, spiritual, and emotional distresses as well.

Evidence of crystals has allegedly been traced back to the legendary city of Atlantis, and there are those who believe that the citizens of Atlantis were gifted in the use of crystals for healing purposes. Crystals have been known to be used for many religious ceremonies in the Native American population as well as in cultures of the Far East. The persistent presence of gemstone therapy throughout history is evidence to the crystal healer that crystals do indeed hold a "magical" healing power.

Philosophy

The theory behind crystal therapy is based on physical properties that some crystals display. (Quartz is the crystal therapists refer to when speaking of crystals in a general sense.) Quartz is composed of silicon dioxide (SiO_2). Natural healers believe that the SiO_2 in the crystal communicates with SiO_2

About This Chapter: "Crystal Therapy" by Anne Bode, M.D. Reprinted with permission from the Creighton University School of Medicine Complementary and Alternative Medicine website, http://altmed.creighton.edu. © 2002 Creighton University School of Medicine.

in the human body. It is this common link that allows energy to transfer from the crystal into the body and promotes healing.

Certain crystals do possess vibrational energy that is known as the piezo-electric effect. This effect does allow crystals to expand with certain frequencies of energy.

The frequency of the vibrational energy released by the crystal is different for every color of gem. Based on this, it is thought that different gemstones, with different vibratory rates, can be used to treat different ailments of the body, mind, spirit, etc.

The human body is made up of many individual parts. These parts have their own unique energy and vibratory rate as well. This energy is emitted to the area surrounding the body. There are seven main energy centers in the body, and these are known as the Chakras. Sickness, stress, and impurities alter the natural frequency of the body, causing some areas of the body to be unable to receive the necessary energy. The body will not be in harmony, and sickness will be overwhelming.

Crystals have pure and constant vibrations; therefore, they are able to "fix" the imbalance in the human body.

Chakras

Chakra is the Sanskrit work for circular motion. A chakra is a spherical energy center that is forever in a fluctuating balance. Physical, emotional, mental, or spiritual blocks can disrupt the energy flowing through a chakra. The energy field of a chakra is affected by everything around us.

> ♣ **It's A Fact!!**
>
> It is believed that the energy given off by crystals is able to balance, clean, and re-energize the energy field of humans.

There are seven main chakras, and they are as follows:

1. **Coccyx (tail bone):** The coccyx chakra resonates with the energy of ontological knowledge, groundedness, presence, and connection with elements around us. The healthy aura emitted by the coccyx is red in

color. There are several gemstones, including red jasper, lapis lazuli, flame agate, ruby, and azurite, whose energies resonate with the coccyx chakra.

2. **Sacrum:** The sacrum chakra resonates with the energy of human emotions, sexuality, creativity and anger, fear, and intuitive knowledge regarding persons, places, and things. The sacrum's healthy aura is orange. The stones resonating with this chakra include opal, fire agate, rose quartz, carnelian, and the actinolite in quartz.

3. **Solar plexus:** The solar plexus chakra is the energy resonance for the power of human will, control and free will, accomplishment, and ego projections. Its healthy aura is yellow in color. Its gemstones of energy resonance are laguna agate, jasper, howlite, amber, morganite, heliodor, and golden citrine.

4. **Heart:** The heart chakra resonates with what it means to be human. Its healthy aura is a radiant green. Its gemstones of energy resonance are emerald, jade, ruby, and plume agate.

5. **Throat:** This chakra is the energy of speech and hearing, self-expression and communication in general, and human intention, definition, and description. Its healthy aura color is indigo blue surrounding clear light. Its resonating energy gemstones are pearl, carnelian, turquoise, bloodstone, malachite, and jasper.

6. **Brow:** The brow chakra is the energy resonance of human inner sight, such as intuition, visions, dreams, charisma, emotional sensitivity, and perception. Its healthy aura emits a deep sea blue. Gemstones resonating with the energy of the brow chakra include sapphire, sugilite, fluorite, azurite, lapis lazuli, opal, iolite, labradorite, and celestite.

7. **Crown (top of the head):** This chakra resonates with the energy of wisdom, spiritual insight, aspirations, and perception of truth. This chakra's healthy aura is ultraviolet surrounding clear light. Gemstones resonating with the crown chakra include moldavite, lepidolite, and danburite.

Gemstones

The following stones are commonly used in crystal therapy. The stone is listed along with its purported effects.

- **Amethyst:** Linked to the mind, amethyst increases hormone production and strengthens the cardiovascular and immune systems, the blood, the metabolism, and the organs of cleansing. It also aids in nerve signaling and transmission and increases memory and communication. Finally, it can aid in the clearing of stomach problems and headaches; the treatment of the eyes, scalp, hair, and pituitary gland; and the decrease of anger and the effects of diabetes.

- **Aquamarine:** Aquamarine calms the body and relieves anxiety while strengthening the cardiovascular, immune, and lymphatic systems.

- **Bloodstone:** Bloodstone strengthens the circulatory system and aids in the detoxification of the kidney, liver, spleen, and blood. It bears a minor influence on the bones, heart, and reproductive organs.

- **Calcite:** Calcite benefits the cleansing organs and the bones and joints. It further sharpens mental clarity and boosts the memory.

- **Carnelian:** Carnelian balances creativity and thoughts. It exercises strengthening effects on the reproductive organs, pancreas, kidneys, and gallbladder. Like bloodstone, it purifies the liver and the blood. Carnelian serves also to soothe lower back pain, arthritic pain and cramps, and it alleviates allergies. It boosts confidence and increases appetite and sexuality.

- **Citrine:** Citrine has the power to alleviate gastroesophageal reflux (GERD) and allergies. Its energy has an uplifting effect and increases problem-solving abilities. It can also correctly align the spine and strengthen the genitourinary and gastrointestinal systems.

- **Clear quartz:** This stone serves to create bodily harmony while purifying it and returning it to its least diseased state.

- **Diamond:** Diamonds increase trust, clarity, prosperity, and love. In addition, they increase energy while treating glaucoma and problems with the brain and the testicles.

- **Emerald:** Emeralds promote physical and emotional health. They are the stones of inspiration, balance, healing, and patience. Emeralds have beneficial effects on blood sugar, childbirth, and the eyes, and they strengthen the thymus, the lymphatics, and the cardio respiratory system.

- **Garnet:** This stone is one of creativity and passion. It also strengthens the cardiovascular system.

- **Ruby:** The ruby decreases the effects of infections, harmful cholesterol, and blood clots. In addition, it allows anger to surface; it decreases impotency and increases vitality, stamina, and leadership. It is also a body purifier, and it strengthens the cardiovascular system.

- **Sapphire:** The sapphire decreases the effects of inflammation/fever, nosebleeds, tuberculosis, burns, tension, depression, and confusion. Sapphire is beneficial in removing foreign bodies from the eye.

Ailments

Ailments and conditions that crystals can cure are myriad. They are as follows:

- Acute pain
- Allergies
- Cancer
- Chronic pain
- Diabetes
- Esophageal problems
- Hormonal problems
- Intestinal problems
- Liver disorders
- Nervous system disorders
- Prostate problems
- Respiratory system problems
- Spleen problems
- AIDS
- Bladder problems
- Circulatory problems
- Depression
- Eating disorders
- Gallbladder problems
- Hypertension
- Kidney disorders
- Lymphatic problems
- Pancreatic problems
- Reproductive system problems
- Spinal disease
- Stomach problems

In addition to curing disease, crystals promote energy levels, induce relaxation, and relieve stress.

Medical/Scientific Information

Skeptics of crystal therapy contend that crystal therapists misunderstand the piezoelectric effect, the very basis of therapists' attribution to crystals of healing power. The piezoelectric effect is the generation of a potential difference across opposite faces of non-conducting crystals as a result of the application of mechanical stress between these faces. In other words, crystals produce an electrical charge when compressed. It is ostensibly this singular characteristic of crystals that has misled New Age crystal therapists into believing that crystals can harness and then direct energy to the benefit of the human body.

The phenomenon of the piezoelectric effect is generated only under very specific conditions in which the particular crystal is cut into extremely thin slices and directed along particular orientations and axes. Furthermore, one should note that most gemstones cannot be made to exhibit the piezoelectric effect. Quartz and tourmaline are among the few gemstones that will demonstrate this phenomenon.

♣ **It's A Fact!!**
There is no actual scientific evidence, only anecdotal support, that crystals are able to conduct any healing energy.

Chapter 41

Enzyme Therapy

Enzyme therapy is a plan of dietary supplements of plant and animal enzymes used to facilitate the digestive process and improve the body's ability to maintain balanced metabolism.

Origins

Enzymes are protein molecules used by the body to perform all of its chemical actions and reactions. The body manufactures several thousands of enzymes. Among them are the digestive enzymes produced by the stomach, pancreas, small intestine, and the salivary glands of the mouth. Their energy-producing properties are responsible for the digestion of nutrients and their absorption, transportation, metabolization, and elimination.

Enzyme therapy is based on the work of Dr. Edward Howell in the 1920s and 1930s. Howell proposed that enzymes from foods work in the stomach to pre-digest food. He advocated the consumption of large amounts of plant enzymes, theorizing that if the body had to use less of its own enzymes for digestion, it could store them for maintaining metabolic harmony. Four categories of plant enzymes are helpful in pre-digestion: protease, amylase, lipase, and cellulase. Cellulase is particularly helpful because the body is unable to produce it.

About This Chapter: Information in this chapter is from "Enzyme Therapy," from *Gale Encyclopedia of Alternative Medicine*, by Mary McNutty and Teresa Olde, Volume 2, Gale Group, © 2005, Thomson/Gale. Reprinted by permission of The Gale Group.

Animal enzymes, such as pepsin extracted from the stomach of pigs, work more effectively in the duodenum. They are typically used for the treatment of non-digestive ailments.

The seven categories of food enzymes and their activities are as follows:

- Amylase: breaks down starches
- Cellulase: breaks down fibers
- Lactase: breaks down dairy products
- Lipase: breaks down fats
- Maltase: breaks down grains
- Protease: breaks down proteins
- Sucrase: breaks down sugars

Enzyme theory generated further interest as the human diet became more dependent on processed and cooked foods. Enzymes are extremely sensitive to heat, and temperatures above 118°F (48°C) destroy them. Modern processes of pasteurization, canning, and microwaving are particularly harmful to the enzymes in food.

Benefits

In traditional medicine, enzyme supplements are often prescribed for patients suffering from disorders that affect the digestive process, such as cystic fibrosis, Gaucher's disease, diabetes, and celiac disease. A program of enzyme supplementation is rarely recommended for healthy patients. However, proponents of enzyme therapy believe that such a program is beneficial for everyone. They point to enzymes' ability to purify the blood, strengthen the immune system, enhance mental capacity, cleanse the colon, and maintain proper pH balance in urine. They feel that by improving the digestive process, the body is better able to combat infection and disease.

Some evidence exists that pancreatic enzymes derived from animal sources are helpful in cancer treatment. The enzymes may be able to dissolve the coating on cancer cells and may make it easier for the immune system to attack the cancer.

In 2002, a biopharmaceutical company received consideration from the U.S. Food and Drug Administration (FDA) to apply for approval of a new enzyme replacement therapy that would provide long-term treatment for patients with Fabry's disease, a condition characterized by defective digestion. Fabry's disease patients don't digest fat properly, and as a result, develop kidney and heart problems in adulthood. The therapy under development is called Replagal (agalsidase alfa).

Description

Enzyme supplements are extracted from plants like pineapple and papaya and from the organs of cows and pigs. The supplements are typically given in tablet or capsule form. Pancreatic enzymes may also be given by injection. The dosage varies with the condition being treated. For non-digestive ailments, the supplements are taken in the hour before meals so

---

✤ It's A Fact!!
Some Complaints And Illnesses That Can Be Treated By Enzyme Therapy

• Acute inflammation	• AIDS
• Alcohol consumption	• Anemia
• Anxiety	• Back pain
• Cancer	• Chronic fatigue syndrome
• Colds	• Colitis
• Constipation	• Diarrhea
• Food allergies	• Gastric duodenal ulcer
• Gastritis	• Gout
• Headaches	• Hepatitis
• Hypoglycemia	• Infections
• Mucous congestion	• Multiple sclerosis
• Nervous disorders	• Nutritional disorders
• Obesity	• Premenstrual syndrome (PMS)
• Stress	

that they can be quickly absorbed into the blood. For digestive ailments, the supplements are taken immediately before meals accompanied by a large glass of fluids. Pancreatic enzymes may be accompanied by doses of vitamin A.

Preparations

No special preparations are necessary before beginning enzyme therapy. However, it is always advisable to talk to a doctor or pharmacist before purchasing enzymes and beginning therapy.

Precautions

People with allergies to beef, pork, pineapples, and papaya may suffer allergic reactions to enzyme supplements. Tablets are often coated to prevent them from breaking down in the stomach, and usually shouldn't be chewed or crushed. People who have difficulty swallowing pills can request enzyme supplements in capsule form. The capsules can then be opened and the contents sprinkled onto soft foods like applesauce.

✎ What's It Mean?

Celiac Disease: A chronic disease characterized by defective digestion and use of fats.

Cystic Fibrosis: A genetic disease that causes multiple digestive, excretion, and respiratory complications. Among the effects, the pancreas fails to provide secretions needed for the digestion of food.

Duodenum: The first part of the small intestine.

Gaucher's Disease: A rare genetic disease caused by a deficiency of enzymes needed for the processing of fatty acids.

Metabolism: The system of chemical processes necessary for living cells to remain healthy.

Side Effects

Side effects associated with enzyme therapy include heartburn, nausea and vomiting, diarrhea, bloating, gas, and acne. According to the principles of therapy, these are temporary cleansing symptoms. Drinking eight to ten glasses of water daily and getting regular exercise can reduce the discomfort of these side effects. Individuals may also experience an increase in bowel movements, perhaps one or two per day. This is also considered a positive effect.

Plant enzymes are safe for pregnant women, although they should always check with a doctor before using enzymes. Pregnant women should avoid animal enzymes. In rare cases, extremely high doses of enzymes can result in a build up of uric acid in the blood or urine and can cause a break down of proteins.

Research And General Acceptance

In the United States, the FDA has classified enzymes as a food. Therefore, they can be purchased without a prescription. However, insurance coverage is usually dependent upon the therapy resulting from a doctor's orders.

Training And Certification

There is no specific training or certification required for practicing enzyme therapy.

Chapter 42

Probiotics

What is a probiotic?

Probiotic literally means "for life." The best way to think of probiotics is as live, microbial cultures consumed or applied for a health benefit. Most probiotic products contain the bacteria from the genera *Lactobacillus* or *Bifidobacterium*, although other genera, including *Escherichia*, *Enterococcus*, and *Saccharomyces* (a yeast) have been marketed as probiotics. Most probiotic products are consumed orally.

Are bacteria bad?

Bacteria are small, single-celled living creatures. Most bacteria are not harmful; in fact, our bodies carry about 100,000,000,000,000 (100 trillion) bacteria, most in our colon. They live and grow there and help prime our immune system so we can better fight infection. There are, however, harmful bacteria that cause infections, even disease. Some bacteria also can produce byproducts from their growth that are associated with cancer. Consuming probiotics is one approach to reducing the impact of harmful bacteria that live in our gastrointestinal tract or that we are exposed to.

About This Chapter: Information in this chapter is from "Frequently Asked Questions & Consumer Information." Reprinted with permission from http://www .USprobiotics.org. © 2004 California Dairy Research Foundation, Dairy & Food Culture Technologies. All rights reserved.

Do healthy people need to add probiotics to their diet?

While people do not require probiotics to be healthy, there is mounting evidence that probiotics can help people stay healthy in certain ways, such as improving immune function, maintaining normal GI function, and preventing infection. Probiotics also have been shown to be effective in management of certain diseases, such as reducing the development of atopic dermatitis in infants or reducing recurrence of pouchitis.

What products contain probiotic bacteria?

Probiotic bacteria have a long history of association with fermented dairy products. If you eat yogurt, you are likely eating probiotics. Some milk contains probiotic bacteria (check the labels). In addition, many dietary supplement products marketed in health food or grocery stores also contain probiotic bacteria.

Which probiotic strain is the right one?

This is a difficult question, since it depends on so many factors. Not all probiotic strains are the same. Different strains of even the same genus or species are not necessarily the same. (For example, two different strains of *Lactobacillus acidophilus* might not have the same probiotic activity.) To better understand this concept, think of dogs. We know that dogs are all the same species, but different breeds of dogs can be very different. A golden retriever may be good for bird hunting while a German shepherd is a good watchdog. It's clear that one breed of dog should not be expected to be right for all purposes. Strains of bacteria are very similar. Some strains of probiotics, even of the same species, can have very different characteristics. That's why it is important to know what exact strain is being used and what documented evidence is available for the specific strain being used. Few probiotic supplement products and no dairy products in the United States list strain designations on product labels for the strains being used. The information on strain identity may be available from the manufacturer.

Unfortunately, some companies know very little about the probiotic strain they are selling. It is very common for companies to cite scientific

Probiotics257

studies conducted on bacteria perhaps related to, but different from, those they are selling in an effort to substantiate efficacy. Scientific studies are expensive to conduct, and many companies have not sponsored them. If studies have not been conducted on a probiotic strain, it is impossible to know for certain if the strain can survive and function as a probiotic in the human body. An undocumented strain might be effective; however, consumers should be aware of the importance of scientific documentation of probiotic efficacy. Your best bet is to purchase a product made by a company you trust and one that can provide documentation of health effects for the specific strains used in their products.

How many probiotic bacteria are contained in the product?

In the case of capsule and other oral supplement formats, probiotic products generally indicate levels of bacteria on the label. In the case of most food products, however, the level of viable bacteria is usually not indicated. Claimed levels of 0.1–10 billion are common in dietary supplement products. In dairy products, generally milk with probiotics contains about 200–300 million per cup. One milk-based product, Dannon's DanActive (Actimel in Europe), contains 10 billion bacteria per serving. A study conducted by consumerlabs.com (http://www.consumerlabs.com/results/probiotics.asp) concluded that one-third of probiotic products do not contain the levels of active bacteria they claim.

It should be noted that some studies surveying commercial products report the use of methods, which do not properly enumerate the probiotic bacteria from products. This can lead to erroneous conclusions about inadequacy of probiotic levels in commercial products, which are actually properly formulated. Unfortunately, no independent, third party organization exists that uses validated methods to certify that probiotic products meet their label claims. Although the Food and Drug Administration requires labeling of foods and supplements to be truthful and not misleading, they do not enforce this by testing.

Do probiotics remain alive throughout shelf life?

Many probiotic bacteria are stable (that is, they remain alive) as dried bacteria (in capsules, for example), especially if kept refrigerated, and in dairy products. Some people think if bacteria are dried, they can't possibly be alive. If bacteria are dried and stabilized properly, they remain alive (while dormant) and start to grow again after they reach the moist environment inside your body. However, stability differs for different strains, different storage conditions and different product formats. Some research studies have shown that probiotic products do not always contain the levels of bacteria they claim or that would be expected in the product. Therefore, it is important to purchase your product from a responsible company. Check with the product manufacturer to confirm levels of live bacteria expected in the product at the end of shelf life. Also, be sure to follow manufacturers' recommendations on how to store the product once purchased.

Are probiotics safe?

In general, probiotics comprised of *Lactobacillus* and *Bifidobacterium* are safe. Some products marketed as probiotics are undefined mixtures of microorganisms of other genera, and it is difficult to know if they are safe or not.

Should I consult with my doctor before taking probiotics? Are there people who should not take probiotics?

It's always a good idea to include your health care professional in any decision about your health. People who are immunocompromised, or have an underlying disease or gut condition, should take probiotics only under the care of a doctor, and even then, should only take well defined and characterized products produced by reputable companies.

How many and how often should probiotics be consumed for an effect?

Most positive clinical studies conducted in humans have used probiotics at high levels, around 10^{9-11} viable cells per day. Unfortunately, most studies have not tested to see if lower levels would be adequate. Many of the studies are conducted on disease endpoints, so often the question of what it takes to keep you healthy (as opposed to what it takes to make you better once sick) is not addressed. Lower levels of probiotics consumed over long periods of time may be adequate for prevention of

✔ Quick Tip
Adding Probiotics To Your Diet

Consumers are often confused about adding probiotics to their diets because it is difficult to know which probiotic product to choose. There is a lot of misinformation, overstatement of scientific results, and just plain misleading positioning of some probiotics products on the market. In order to reap the health benefits they have to offer, you need to consume an adequate level of viable probiotics. Unfortunately, many probiotic foods and/or supplements either do not indicate the level of probiotics contained in them or they report levels of probiotics on their label that are not maintained throughout the shelf life of the product.

If you are interested in a product, call the manufacturer and ask the following questions:

• What health benefits have been documented for your specific probiotic product?

• Remember to ask for specific reference citations or copies of the articles that have been published. See if they are general review articles or articles pertaining to the specific strains of bacteria used in the product. General review articles are interesting but not relevant to the specific formulation being sold.

• What levels of all probiotics contained in the product are present at the end of the shelf life (assuming appropriate storage conditions)?

• Does the company regularly survey their product to know that it meets the label claims once it is on the shelf?

• Does the company use an objective, independent laboratory to certify that their product meets label claims?

Once you have decided on a specific product, pay attention to how it works for you. Keep in mind that we all have a unique physiology, different composition of our native flora, and distinctive nutritional status. We each might respond differently to different formulations. If a product works for you, stick with it. If, after one month, a product does not work for you, try something else.

some illness. In addition, it may depend on the specific probiotic strain you are taking. The ability of a strain to survive through the stomach and into the intestine is different for different strains. Generalizations to all probiotic products are difficult to make. The product manufacturer should be able to tell you what levels have been shown to be effective for the strains they are selling.

How will probiotics affect my health?

Some probiotic bacteria consumed orally have been shown to improve the digestion of lactose, decrease the incidence and duration of diarrheal illness, and improve immune system function. Their ability to decrease the risk of colon tumors has been documented in animal studies and is currently the subject of a large clinical trial in the European Union. Controlled clinical studies have defined a role for probiotics in the prevention of allergy development in infants at risk for atopic dermatitis and for extending periods of remission of patients with inflammatory bowel disease. Probiotic products may provide special benefit to aging consumers and to people faced with challenging life situations such as stress, antibiotic treatment or travel. People dealing with recurring gastrointestinal symptoms or vaginal infections could discuss with their doctors if probiotics may be useful to try. Of course, not all probiotics will work for all people or for all conditions. One pragmatic approach is to try the product for a month, and see if it helps.

Are probiotics better when you get them from foods or from pills?

Probiotics from foods or pills can be effective. The important consideration is that you are getting high enough numbers of a strain or combination of strains that works for you. Food sources of probiotics have the advantage in that they offer good nutrition along with the probiotic bacteria. Food sources of probiotics, however, are generally lower in potency than supplements. One exception is DanActive (www.danactive.com), a product by Dannon. Other foods may provide high levels of probiotics; but, as they do not state probiotics levels on their labels, it is difficult to know. Supplements can be more convenient for some people and may provide higher levels of probiotic, depending on the specific products.

> **✔ Quick Tip**
> **Guidelines For Selecting A Probiotics Product**
>
> • If you have a specific reason for wanting to take a probiotic (i.e., you suffer from antibiotic associated diarrhea), find a company you trust and ask them for information specific to their product that supports effectiveness for your condition at the dose used in the product.
>
> • If you are interested in probiotics for the general health value of supplementing your diet with beneficial bacteria, consider food sources. That way you are getting the nutrition of the food as well as possible benefits of beneficial microbes.
>
> • Generally, you will be more likely to benefit from a more potent dose than a weaker one.
>
> • Although it sounds contradictory, keep in mind that just because a specific probiotic product has not been tested for a particular condition, it still may be effective. If your only option is to try a product not tested for your condition, try it for one month. If it does not help you in that time period, try a different product or quit.
>
> • If you are being treated for an illness or condition, let your healthcare provider know you are taking, or planning on taking, probiotics. That way, if there is any complication, they know to look for a possible probiotic link.
>
> • Probiotics are not for everyone. If you are immunocompromised or recovering from surgery, be sure to only take probiotics under the advice of a healthcare provider.

Is it possible to increase the good bacteria in your gut without taking probiotics?

Yes. Probiotics—carbohydrates that are not digested by us, but are digested by some beneficial bacteria in the colon—can increase the levels or activities of beneficial bacteria in the gut. In the U.S., probiotics are in some yogurts—Horizon and Stonyfield both include a probiotic. Also, eating raw fruits and vegetables will increase the number of live bacteria you consume—we just don't know for sure how beneficial these uncharacterized bacteria might be.

Are dried bacteria still alive?

Yes. If properly dried, stabilized, and stored, bacteria can remain quite healthy for long periods of time after drying. They regain activity when they encounter the moist regions in your body.

Are dead bacteria as effective as live ones?

Some recent publications have suggested that dead bacteria can have positive physiological effects. In fact, there are commercial products available in other countries that specifically are comprised of dead bacteria. Since probiotics by definition are alive, such products are not probiotics. The number of studies on dead bacteria is quite few, and it is unlikely that dead bacteria could mediate the many positive effects demonstrated by live, probiotic bacteria.

Chapter 43

Magnetic Therapy

The History Of Magnetic Therapy

The use of magnets in medicine has a long and interesting history. Magnetic therapy can be traced back to the 15th century. Paracelsus, a Swiss physician, used natural magnets, "lodestones," to leach diseases such as epilepsy, diarrhea, and hemorrhage from the body. His reasoning was that since magnets could attract iron, maybe they could attract disease from the body.

Permanent carbon-steel magnets were developed in the 1700s, prompting renewed interest in their curative abilities. Franz Mesmer set up a popular Parisian salon where he used his magnets to cure imbalances in "animal magnetism." A Royal Commission was established by Louis XVI to study the validity of "animal magnetism" and found that any benefit brought about by Mesmer's magnets was due to suggestion, not magnetism. Though his claims of healing were debunked, magnetic therapy still remained popular among laypeople. Some of Mesmer's followers became the forefathers of hypnotherapy (thus the root of the word "mesmerize").

In 1799, an American physician, Elisha Perkins, promoted the use of "metallic tractors" to "draw off the noxious electrical fluid that lay at the foot

About This Chapter: Excerpted from "Magnetic Therapy," with permission from the Creighton University School of Medicine Complementary and Alternative Medicine website, http://altmed.creighton.edu. © 2005 Creighton University School of Medicine.

of suffering." Small, wedge-shaped magnets were swept over the ailing person's body and were believed by many to be effective in curing a variety of diseases.

About 100 years after Mesmer, Daniel David Palmer took an interest in magnets and opened Palmer's School of Magnetic Cure in Davenport, Iowa in the last years of the 19th century. Dr. Palmer's philosophy of healing through physical manipulation developed into chiropractic medicine.

Magnetic products were available for purchase from the Sears catalog in the late 1800s. Dr. C. J. Thatcher had his own 1866 catalog, which sold a variety of magnetic devices, including a suit with over 700 magnets, which offered complete magnetic protection. He reported that magnetism, properly applied, could cure virtually any ailment.

In the 20th century, newer and stronger magnets were developed: alnico magnets in the 1930s, ferrite (ceramic) magnets in the 1950s, and rare earth metal magnets in the 1970s and 1980s. These new magnets have been important in technology and industry and also have sparked renewed interest in the use of magnets in medicine.

Magnetic Therapy Benefit Claims

Many claims are made regarding the benefits due to the application of permanent magnets. Some of the claims are listed below. Properly applied permanent magnets may claim to do the following:

- Increase the blood flow to the area to which they are applied

- Reduce pain

- Decrease inflammation

- Speed recovery of bone fractures

- Shrink tumors or cure cancer

Magnetic devices are available in a variety of products. Most of them contain small disks of ferrite or rare earth magnets arranged differently according to the philosophy of the manufacturer. "Multi-polar" devices have magnets arranged in an alternating north/south pattern, whereas "uni-polar" magnets have only one pole facing the patient. The magnets may be arranged in circular, triangular, or checkerboard patterns. Some manufacturers claim that only south-seeking poles facing the body should be used, since south-seeking poles have a calming effect on tissues, therefore, would reduce inflammation, infection, and pain, and would shrink tumors. Evidently, in the southern hemisphere, north-seeking poles are used instead to calm tissues.

Products that are available range from magnetic pads (shoe insoles, small Band-Aid-like patches, or wraps which may be applied to virtually any part of the body) to magnetic jewelry, to magnetic bed accessories.

Some Discussion Regarding Magnetic Therapy

There is no known scientific reason that permanent magnets applied to the skin would cause any recognizable physiological effect. Further research needs to be undertaken to understand what, if any, effect permanent magnets has in humans.

It was mentioned earlier that magnet manufacturers use patient testimonials to sell magnetic devices. Why do so many people claim that magnets were helpful in relieving their pain? The placebo effect can be a powerful influence on patients. Simply stated, positive effects are seen in patients who are administered inactive substances, that is, placebos. Paracelsus, one of the first physicians to use magnets therapeutically, wrote, "the spirit is the master, the imagination is the instrument, the body is the plastic material. The moral atmosphere surrounding the patient can have a strong influence on the course of the disease. It is not the curse or the blessing that works, but the idea. The imagination produces the effect." Evidently, Paracelsus was aware of the placebo effect. Thirty percent of patients are commonly found to respond positively to placebos. The reason for studies, which are placebo-controlled, is to recognize the placebo effect and to take it into account in the analysis of data.

It seems that there are no harmful effects from using magnets, but is there any real benefit? It is true that very few scientifically valid experiments have been undertaken to assess the possible benefit of magnets in the treatment of pain.

Magnets And Depression

Depression affects over 37 million people per year. It is an illness that is oftentimes managed quite nicely through a wide array of medical, psychiatric, and alternative therapies. Despite the impressive arsenal, it is estimated that 10% of those people who suffer from depression are refractory to conventional forms of treatment. The many people who remain refractory to treatment are left with few alternatives to this life altering illness.

Alternatives to conventional medical management of depression includes psychotherapy (including interpersonal and group therapies), electroconvulsive therapy (ECT), and light therapy. In recent years use of transcranial magnetic stimulation (TMS) has been studied and is showing promise to those who suffer from severe refractory depression.

During TMS procedure, which lasts only about 5 minutes, the patient sits comfortably in a chair while a strong magnetic field (100–1000 Gauss) is applied transcranially in short bursts of one-second duration.

✎ What's It Mean?

Electroconvulsive Therapy (ECT): Uses low voltage electrical stimulation of the brain to treat some forms of major depression, acute mania, and some forms of schizophrenia. This potentially life-saving technique is considered only when other therapies have failed, when a person is seriously medically ill and/or unable to take medication, or when a person is very likely to commit suicide. Substantial improvements in the equipment, dosing guidelines, and anesthesia have significantly reduced the possibility of side effects. [1]

Light Therapy: Involves the use of artificial light to simulate sunlight. [2]

Refractory: Not responsive to treatment. [3]

Source: [1] "Mental Health Dictionary," National Mental Health Information Center, Substance Abuse and Mental Health Services Administration, cited April 2006. [2] "Seasonal Depression Awareness Month," National Mental Health Information Center, Substance Abuse and Mental Health Services Administration, December 2003. [3] Editor.

The magnet is placed over the left froto-temporal lobe. The procedure is very safe and provides little risk for side effects, especially when compared to ECT. Some patients describe the procedure as a small tapping sensation on the skull.

✔ Quick Tip

Without further evidence to support their benefit, consumers should avoid spending a lot of money on magnetic devices for the relief of pain.

Source: © 2005 Creighton University School of Medicine.

In June of 2000, Pridmore et. al. published in the *International Journal of Neuropsychopharmacology* a study comparing the outcomes of repetitive transcranial magnetic stimulation (rTMS) to that of electroconvulsive therapy. The study size was small, but the rate of remission between the two treatment modalities was equal. While ECT was found to diminish the severity of the depression through the course of the treatment at a higher rate than rTMS, the numbers were not found to be statistically significant.

In July 2002, an article published in the *American Journal of Psychiatry* by Hoffman et al. found exciting evidence that suggested slow, repetitive transcranial magnetic stimulation reduces cortical activity, thereby reducing symptoms of patients enrolled in preliminary trials such as dystonia, seizures, and auditory hallucinations.

While magnets continue to be a multi-billion dollar business in the management of chronic pain while showing little scientific evidence they perform better than placebo, preliminary evidence for their ability to assist with treatment resistant depression is encouraging and continues to be studied.

Chapter 44

Reiki

Where does Reiki energy come from?

Reiki energy is a subtle energy. It is different than electricity or chemical energy or other kinds of physical energy. Reiki energy comes from the Higher Power, which exists on a higher dimension than the physical world we are familiar with. When viewed clairvoyantly, Reiki energy appears to come down from above and to enter the top of the practitioner's head after which it flows through the body and out the hands. It appears to flow this way because of our perspective. However, the true source of Reiki energy is within us. This does not mean that we use our personal energy when we do Reiki, but that the energy is coming from a transcendental part of ourselves that is connected to an infinite supply of healing energy.

Is Reiki a religion?

Although Reiki energy is spiritual in nature, Reiki is not a religion. Practitioners are not asked to change any religious or spiritual beliefs they may have. They are free to continue believing anything they choose and are encouraged to make their own decisions concerning the nature of their religious practices.

How is a Reiki treatment given?

In a standard treatment, Reiki energy flows from the practitioner's hands into the client. The client is usually lying on a massage table, but treatments can also be given while the client is seated or even standing. The client remains fully clothed. The practitioner places her/his hands on or near the client's body in a series of hand positions. These include positions around the head and shoulders, the stomach, and feet. Other, more specific positions may be used based on the clients needs. Each position is held for three to ten minutes depending on how much Reiki the client needs at each position. The whole treatment usually lasts between 45 and 90 minutes.

What does a Reiki treatment feel like?

What one experiences during a Reiki treatment varies somewhat from person to person. However, all usually feel feelings of deep relaxation. In addition, many feel a wonderful glowing radiance that flows through and surrounds them. As the Reiki energy encourages one to let go of all tension, anxiety, fear, or other negative feelings, a state of peace and well-being is experienced. Some drift off to sleep or report floating outside their bodies or have visions and other mystical experiences. At the end of the treatment, one feels refreshed with a more positive, balanced outlook.

What can be treated with Reiki?

Reiki has had a positive affect on all forms of illness and negative conditions. This includes minor things like head or stomachaches, bee stings, colds, flu, tension, and anxiety as well as serious illness like heart disease, cancer, leukemia, etc. The side effects of regular medical treatments have also been reduced or eliminated. This includes the negative effects of chemotherapy, post-operative pain, and depression as well as improving the healing rate and reducing the time needed to stay in the hospital. Reiki always helps, and in some cases, people have experienced complete healings, which have been confirmed by medical tests before and after the Reiki treatments. However, while some have experienced miracles, they cannot be guaranteed. Stress reduction with some improvement in ones physical and psychological condition are what most experience.

Does one have to stop seeing a regular doctor or psychologist in order to receive a Reiki treatment?

No. Reiki works in conjunction with regular medical or psychological treatment. Reiki energy works in harmony with all other forms of healing including drugs, surgery, psychological care or any other method of alternative care, and will improve the results.

Who can learn to do Reiki?

Reiki is a very simple technique to learn and is not dependent on one having any prior experience with healing, meditation or any other kind of training. Over one million people from all walks of life, both young and old, have successfully learned it. The reason it is so easy to learn is that it is not taught in the usual way something is taught. The ability to do Reiki is simply transferred from the teacher to the student through a process called an attunement that takes place during a Reiki class. As soon as one receives an attunement, they have the ability to do Reiki, and after that, whenever one places their hands on themselves or on another person with the intention of doing Reiki, the healing energy will automatically begin flowing.

How long does it take to learn Reiki?

A beginning Reiki class is taught on a weekend. The class can be one or two days long. It is recommended that the minimum time necessary be at least six to seven hours. Along with the attunement, it is necessary that the student be shown how to give treatments and also to practice giving treatments in class.

What is a Reiki attunement?

A Reiki attunement is the process by which a person receives the ability to give Reiki treatments. The Reiki master administers the attunement during the Reiki class. During the attunement, the Reiki master will touch the student's head, shoulders, and hands and use one or more special breathing techniques. The attunement energies will flow through the Reiki master and into the student. These special energies are guided by the Higher Power and make adjustments in the student's energy pathways and connect the student to the source of Reiki. Because the Higher Power guides the energetic aspect of the attunement, it adjusts itself to be exactly right for each student. During the attunement, some students feel warmth in the hands; others may see colors or have visions of spiritual beings. However, it is not necessary to have an inner experience for the attunement to have worked. Most simply feel more relaxed.

Can I treat myself?

Yes. Once you have received the attunement, you can treat yourself as well as others. This is one of the unique features of Reiki.

I have heard that Reiki can be sent to others at a distance. How does this work?

Yes. In Reiki II, you are given three Reiki symbols. These symbols are empowered by the Reiki II attunement. One of these symbols is for distant healing. By using a picture of the person you would like to send Reiki to or by writing the person's name on a piece of paper or simply by thinking of the person and also activating the distant symbol, you can send Reiki to them no matter where they are. They could be hundreds of miles away, but it makes no difference. The Reiki energy will go to them and treat them. You can also send Reiki to crisis situations or world leaders and the Reiki energy will help them too.

What does it feel like to give a treatment?

When giving a Reiki treatment, the Reiki energy flows through the practitioner before leaving the hands and flowing into the client. Because of this, the practitioner receives a treatment also. As the Reiki energy flows through the practitioner, she/he will feel more relaxed and uplifted. Spiritual experiences sometimes take place. The practitioner sometimes receives insights about what the client needs to know to heal more deeply.

☞ Remember!!
If one has a medical or psychological condition, it is recommended that one see a licensed health care professional in addition to receiving Reiki treatments.

How do I find a Reiki teacher that is right for me?

Reiki teachers or masters advertise in many magazines and also post notices at health food stores, new age bookstores, and other places. Once you find a Reiki teacher or practitioner you are interested in receiving training or a treatment from, it is a good idea to ask them some questions.

Is it safe for pregnant women?

Since Reiki is guided by the Higher Power, the Reiki energy will know the condition of the client or student and adjust appropriately. Reiki can only do good. Many pregnant women have received treatments with great benefit to them and their unborn child. It has also been used during childbirth. Pregnant women have also taken the Reiki training and received the Reiki attunement with beneficial results.

What about babies?

Babies love Reiki. It is very healthy for them. Do not worry about it being too strong. Reiki automatically adjusts to what the baby needs.

Can I treat animals or plants?

Animals love Reiki too. They seem to have a natural understanding of what Reiki is and its benefits. Once a pet has received a Reiki treatment, they will often let you know that they want more. Plants also respond well to Reiki.

Are there any side effects from a Reiki treatment?

Most of the time a person will feel relaxed and uplifted by a Reiki treatment. However, sometimes a person will have what is called a healing crisis. As a person's vibration goes up, toxins that have been stored in the body will be released into the blood stream to be filtered by the liver and kidneys and removed from the system. When this happens, sometimes a person can get a headache or stomachache or feel weak. If this happens, it is a good idea to drink more water, eat lighter meals, and get more rest. The body is cleansing as part of the healing process so this is a good sign.

Can it be used to help groups of people or even global crises?

Yes. This is one of the wonderful benefits of Reiki and is why it is such a wonderful technique for the new millennium. It allows individuals and groups to do something positive about the challenging situations we see on the news involving so many people all over the planet. Reiki can be used to reduce suffering and help people anywhere in the world. As more and more people send Reiki to help the world heal, we will move quickly to a world of peace and harmony.

✔ Quick Tip
Important Questions To Ask Before
Choosing A Reiki Teacher

- How long have you been working with Reiki? What training have you had? How often do you teach? How do you personally use Reiki? What is your lineage?

- What qualifications are required to take Reiki training?

- What do you cover in your classes? How many hours of class time is included? How much time is instructional, and how much is hands on practice?

- What are the specific things I will be able to do after taking the training?

- What are your fees, and will I get a certificate and a manual?

- Can I take notes and tape record the class?

- How many symbols will I learn?

- Is there a Reiki support group in my area or can you help me establish one?

- Will you openly support me in being a successful Reiki practitioner or Master?

- Do you have a positive respectful attitude toward other Reiki practitioners and Masters regardless of lineage or affiliation?

Be aware of how you feel about their answers and if they are responding in a loving manner that is supportive and empowering. Listen to your heart and you will be guided to the right teacher or practitioner.

How much does a treatment usually cost?

A Reiki treatment usually will cost between $25.00 and $100.00 depending on the area of the country. However, some practitioners offer treatments free of charge or for a donation.

Does insurance cover Reiki treatments?

Reiki is just starting to be recognized by insurance companies. While not many are covering Reiki treatments, some are. Check with your insurance company for details.

Can you get more than one attunement?

Once you receive a Reiki attunement, it will last your whole life. However, if you get additional attunements for the same level, it will act to refine and strengthen your Reiki energy.

What is lineage?

Reiki is a technique that is passed on from teacher to student over and over. If one has Reiki, then she/he will be part of a secession of teachers leading back to the founder of the system of Reiki one is practicing.

Chapter 45

Therapeutic Touch

What is therapeutic touch?

Therapeutic touch is a form of healing that uses a practice called "laying on of hands" to correct or balance energy fields. The word "touch" is misleading because there is generally no direct physical touch involved. Instead, the hands are moved just over the body. Therapeutic touch is based on the theory that the body, mind, and emotions form a complex energy field. According to therapeutic touch, health is an indication of a balanced energy field and illness represents imbalance. Studies suggest that therapeutic touch can help to heal wounds, reduce pain, and promote relaxation.

What is the energy field?

Although scientists have not detected a human energy field, the concept of an energy field is also a part of other types of healing. In the ancient medical systems of India and China, the energy field is described as life energy. It is thought to exist throughout the body and is responsible for maintaining normal physiological, psychological, and spiritual functions. In traditional Chinese medicine this energy is called qi (pronounced "chee"), and in India's Ayurvedic medicine it is called prana.

What is the history of therapeutic touch?

Dolores Krieger, a professor at New York University School of Nursing, and Dora Kunz, a natural healer, developed therapeutic touch in the early 1970s. At first, Krieger and Kunz only taught the techniques to Krieger's graduate school nursing students, but Krieger's professional research and writing increased the popularity of the technique, particularly among nurses. The practice grew primarily through a grassroots effort of nurses throughout the United States.

How does therapeutic touch work?

Scientists are not certain how therapeutic touch works. There are few studies, and scientific investigators have so far not detected the human energy field. Still, two theories have been put forward.

One theory is that the actual pain associated with a physically or emotionally painful experience (such as infection, injury, or a difficult relationship) remains in the body's cells. The pain stored in the cells is disruptive and prevents some cells from working properly with other cells in the body. This results in disease. Therapeutic touch is thought to restore health by restoring communication between cells.

The other theory is based on the principles of quantum physics. As blood, which contains iron, circulates in our bodies, an electromagnetic field is produced. According to this theory, at one time we could all easily see this field (called an aura), but now only certain individuals, such as those who practice therapeutic touch, develop this ability.

More generally, therapeutic touch is based on the idea that optimal health requires a balanced flow of life energy. Practitioners of therapeutic touch, by their own description, sense your energy through their hands and then send healthy energy back to you. When receiving therapeutic touch you usually feel such things as warmth, relaxation, and/or pain relief. The practitioner describes your energy as hot or cold, active or passive, blocked or free. There are eight general regions of the body above which energy is sensed—head, throat, heart, stomach, lower abdomen, sacral region, knees, and feet. Ultimately, you, the recipient of therapeutic touch, are the healer. The practitioner simply allows your body's own healing mechanisms to emerge. The role of the practitioner is to facilitate this process.

✤ It's A Fact!!

Therapeutic touch is taught at more than 100 hospitals and health centers worldwide and is most commonly practiced by nurses.

What should I expect on my first visit?

Before the session begins, you will be asked to sit or lie down. No undressing is necessary. Despite its name, therapeutic touch rarely involves physical contact between the therapist and the person being treated. Sessions can be broken down into four steps, which are as follows:

1. **Centering:** The therapist becomes "centered" by using breathing, imagery, and meditation to achieve an altered state of consciousness for him or herself.

2. **Assessment:** The therapist holds his or her hands 2 to 4 inches away from your body while moving from your head to your feet. This is done to assess the energy field surrounding your body. Therapists often describe feelings of warmth, coolness, static, and tingling over the areas of energy "congestion" or "blockage."

3. **Intervention:** Once a congested or blocked area is located, the therapist will move his or her hands in a rhythmic motion starting at the top of the blocked area and moving down and away from your body. This action, known as unruffling, is repeated until the therapist no longer senses congestion or until you begin to sense relief. The therapist will also visualize and transmit life energy to specific areas of your body, which is also intended to correct imbalances.

4. **Evaluation/Closure:** Once you've had a few minutes to relax, the therapist will ask you how you feel. He or she may recheck your energy field to be sure that no blockages were overlooked.

What is therapeutic touch good for?

Most studies indicate that therapeutic touch can relieve tension headaches and reduce pain, such as that associated with burns, osteoarthritis, or following surgery. It may also speed the healing of wounds and improve function in those with arthritis.

Therapeutic touch also promotes relaxation. Cancer, heart disease, and burn patients have reported that therapeutic touch significantly lessens their anxiety. Generally, the deep relaxation associated with therapeutic touch reduces stress, lowers blood pressure, and improves breathing. Being relaxed may also lead to lower cholesterol levels and also may improve immune and bowel functions. Difficult pregnancies may also be made a little easier with the help of therapeutic touch.

Together with medical treatment, therapeutic touch can help with many additional conditions such as the following:

- fibromyalgia

- sleep apnea

- restless leg syndrome (a disorder that causes insomnia)

- allergies

- bronchitis

- addictions

- lupus

- Alzheimer's disease and, possibly, other forms of dementia

> ♣ **It's A Fact!!**
>
> There is controversy as to whether the healing power of therapeutic touch has anything to do with the "laying on of hands." Critics suggest that the healing observed after therapeutic touch may be the result of the relaxing nature of the therapy itself and not the energy transfer that is believed to occur between the therapist's hands and the individual's body.

Some people indicate that they experience emotional and spiritual changes after receiving therapeutic touch. These may include greater self-confidence, self-control, and self-understanding.

Is there anything I should watch out for?

You may feel thirsty, lightheaded, and a need to urinate. Lightheadedness generally only lasts for 15 minutes after a session, but you may feel thirsty for days. According to some practitioners, if you were flooded with too much energy you might feel increased pain and be irritable, restless, anxious, or even nauseated. Therapeutic touch may also worsen fevers and active inflammation; therefore, it is best not to obtain therapeutic touch when you have either a fever or active inflammation (such as an acutely swollen joint from arthritis).

Some therapeutic touch practitioners recommend that children, the elderly, and very sick people be treated for only a short time. Although there is no actual touching involved with therapeutic touch, talk with your practitioner about what to expect from a session, particularly if you have been physically or sexually abused in your past.

How can I find a qualified practitioner?

There is no formal certification program in the United States for therapeutic touch. Most therapeutic touch practitioners are in the nursing profession (although some massage therapists, physical therapists, chiropractors, acupuncturists, and others practice therapeutic touch as well). Nurse Healers-Professional Associates International (NH-PAI) recommends that people look for therapists who practice regularly (at least an average of 2 times per week), have at least 5 years of experience, and have completed at least 12 hours of therapeutic touch workshops.

What is the future of therapeutic touch?

While there appear to be many potential uses for therapeutic touch, particularly for chronically ill people, measuring the effectiveness of the technique is very difficult. Because of this, much of the research that exists has been criticized. Improved studies may lead to wider acceptance.

Part Seven

Using The Senses And Emotions To Enhance Well-Being

Chapter 46

Aromatherapy

Aromatherapy is the therapeutic use of essential oils made from plants and flowers. It is a healing art that aims to rejuvenate body, mind, and spirit. The different smells (aromas), and the chemical constituents of the oils, are said to produce different emotional and physiological reactions. Essential oils can be massaged into the skin, added to bath water, or vaporized in an oil burner. Although aromatherapy has been practiced in some form or another in various cultures for thousands of years, the modern version was developed mainly in France. Aromatherapy has not yet undergone the same scientific scrutiny as other complementary therapies, but research so far shows that it can be an effective treatment for some complaints. Used in a professional way, aromatherapy has little or no negative effects.

A Range Of Symptoms

Aromatherapy is of great benefit as a form of preventative health care. It detoxifies the body, increases blood circulation, and boosts the immune system and the lymphatic system. The oils stimulate, balance, uplift, soothe, and calm. The release of stress and tension can allow the body's own healing process to begin.

About This Chapter: Information in this chapter is from "Aromatherapy." This information was provided by the Better Health Channel. Material on the Better Health Channel is regularly updated. For the latest version of this information, please visit: http://www.betterhealth.vic.gov.au.

Aromatherapy is used to treat a range of disorders, which include the following:

- Digestive problems
- Eczema
- Headaches
- Insomnia
- Stress

Using Essential Oils

Most essential oils are extracted from plant material using steam or water distillation. Selected plant materials are heated with steam, water, or both until the essential oil vaporizes. The oil then condenses as it cools.

All essential oils are concentrated and potent. They should be used very sparingly, only a few drops at a time, and always diluted in some other medium, such as plain massage oil (cold pressed vegetable oil) or unscented base cream (not a mineral oil cream, such as Sorbolene). If essential oils are used undiluted they can cause burning and irritation. Essential oils do not dissolve in water unless mixed with a dispersant first. Some of the ways in which essential oils can be used include the following:

- **Massage:** a small amount added to a vegetable-based oil

- **Oil burner:** a few drops mixed with water and vaporized in a burner

- **Bath:** half a dozen drops added to a full bath

- **Inhalation:** two to three drops added to a basin of hot water

The Sense Of Smell

The nostrils open up inside the skull to form the nasal cavity, which sits directly beneath the brain. Embedded in the ceiling of the nasal cavity are the olfactory cells. Each cell has tiny, moist hairs that trap odor molecules. It is thought that an odor is translated into electrical impulses by these cells, and then passed on to the brain via the two olfactory bulbs. The message is interpreted by a part of the brain called the cerebral cortex. The sense of smell is poorly understood, but we do know that it is linked to the oldest, most primitive part of our brain and seems to have a direct link to our emotions.

Change Is Triggered In The Brain

According to aromatherapy theory, the essential oil molecules bring about changes in the brain. These brain changes, in turn, bring about alterations in various body systems, such as digestion or blood pressure. Some researchers believe that when people experience mood changes or physical changes, it is because the smell has triggered a memory. For instance, if a person feels relaxed when they smell cinnamon, it might be because cinnamon conjures up pleasant childhood memories. However, practitioners maintain that inhaling an essential oil will usually trigger a predictable response, even if the person does not have any memories associated with the smell.

Some Examples Of Popular Aromatherapy Oils

A few of the popular aromatherapy oils and their uses include the following:

- **Peppermint:** digestive disorders

- **Rosemary:** muscular pains, mental stimulant

- **Sandalwood:** depression, anxiety, and nervous tension

- **Tea tree:** respiratory problems, anti-fungal, anti-bacterial, and anti-viral

- **Lavender:** headaches, insomnia, burns, aches, and pains

Special Considerations

People with certain conditions, such as high blood pressure, epilepsy, and pregnancy, should avoid some oils.

Pregnancy

Oils to avoid during pregnancy include the following:

- Basil
- Cedarwood
- Clary sage
- Cypress
- Fennel
- Jasmine
- Juniper
- Sweet marjoram
- Myrrh
- Peppermint
- Rosemary
- Sage
- Thyme

Epilepsy

Oils to avoid with epilepsy include the following:

- Fennel
- Hyssop
- Sage

High Blood Pressure

Oils to avoid with high blood pressure include the following:

- Hyssop
- Rosemary
- Sage
- Thyme

Some People May Be Sensitive To Essential Oils

Some oils can irritate or burn the skin, while others can bring on an allergic reaction, such as a skin rash, in susceptible people. Some of the oils that may cause problems include the following:

- Eucalyptus
- Ginger
- Thyme
- Black pepper
- Cinnamon
- Clove
- Oregano
- Lemongrass
- Some citrus oils

Handle With Care

Some essential oils are toxic and should never be used at all—for example, camphor, pennyroyal, and wintergreen. Essential oils are very potent and should never be swallowed or applied undiluted to the skin. People with asthma and those prone to nose bleeds should use caution when inhaling vaporizing oils.

Where To Get Help

- Qualified professional aromatherapy practitioner
- Doctors or naturopaths with aromatherapy training

> ☞ **Remember!!**
>
> - Aromatherapy is the use of essential oils to bring about physiological and emotional changes.
>
> - The limited research done so far indicates that aromatherapy is helpful for a number of disorders, such as stress-related complaints.
>
> - Essential oils should never be swallowed or applied undiluted to the skin.

Chapter 47

Art Therapy

What is art therapy?

Art therapy is an established mental health profession that uses the creative process of art making to improve and enhance the physical, mental, and emotional well being of individuals of all ages. It is based on the belief that the creative process involved in artistic self-expression helps people to resolve conflicts and problems, develop interpersonal skills, manage behavior, reduce stress, increase self-esteem and self-awareness, and achieve insight.

Art therapy integrates the fields of human development, visual art (drawing, painting, sculpture, and other art forms), and the creative process with models of counseling and psychotherapy. Art therapy is used with children, adolescents, adults, older adults, groups, and families to assess and treat the following: anxiety, depression, and other mental and emotional problems and disorders; mental illness; substance abuse and other addictions; family and relationship issues; abuse and domestic violence; social and emotional difficulties related to disability and illness; trauma and loss; physical, cognitive, and neurological problems; and psychosocial difficulties related to medical

About This Chapter: Information in this chapter is from "About Art Therapy" and "Frequently Asked Questions About Art Therapy." © 2006 American Art Therapy Association, Inc. Reprinted with permission of the American Art Therapy Association, Inc., 5999 Stevenson Avenue, Alexandria, VA 22304, www.arttherapy.org.

illness. Art therapy programs are found in a number of settings including hospitals, clinics, public and community agencies, wellness centers, educational institutions, businesses, and private practices.

What are the qualifications of an art therapist?

Art therapists are master's level professionals who hold a degree in art therapy or a related field. Educational requirements include: theories of art therapy, counseling, and psychotherapy; ethics and standards of practice; assessment and evaluation; individual, group, and family techniques; human and creative development; multicultural issues; research methods; and practicum experiences in clinical, community, and/or other settings. Art therapists are skilled in the application of a variety of art modalities (drawing, painting, sculpture, and other media) for assessment and treatment.

How did art therapy begin?

Visual expression has been used for healing throughout history, but art therapy did not emerge as a distinct profession until the 1940s. In the early 20th century, psychiatrists became interested in the artwork created by their patients with mental illness. At around the same time, educators were discovering that children's art expressions reflected developmental, emotional, and cognitive growth. By mid-century, hospitals, clinics, and rehabilitation centers increasingly began to include art therapy programs along with traditional "talk therapies," underscoring the recognition that the creative process of art making enhanced recovery, health, and wellness. As a result, the profession of art therapy grew into an effective and important method of communication, assessment, and treatment with children and adults in a variety of settings.

Where do art therapists work?

Art therapists work in a wide variety of settings, including, but not limited to, the following:

- Hospitals and clinics, both medical and psychiatric

> ## ♣ It's A Fact!!
> The field of art therapy has gained attention in health care facilities throughout the United States and within psychiatry, psychology, counseling, education, and the arts.
>
> Source: "Frequently Asked Questions About Art Therapy." © 2006 American Art Therapy Association, Inc.

- Outpatient mental health agencies and day treatment facilities

- Residential treatment centers

- Halfway houses

- Domestic violence and homeless shelters

- Community agencies and non-profit settings

- Sheltered workshops

- Schools, colleges, and universities

- Correctional facilities

- Elder care facilities

- Art studios

- Private practice

An art therapist may work as part of a team that includes physicians, psychologists, nurses, mental health counselors, marriage and family therapists, rehabilitation counselors, social workers, and teachers. Together, they determine and implement a client's therapeutic goals and objectives. Other art therapists work independently and maintain private practices with children, adolescents, adults, groups, and/or families.

Chapter 48

Dance Therapy

Dance is the most fundamental of the arts, involving direct expression through the body. Thus, it is an intimate and powerful medium for therapy. Based on the assumption that body and mind are interrelated, dance/movement therapy is defined by the American Dance Therapy Association as "the psychotherapeutic use of movement as a process which furthers the emotional, cognitive and physical integration of the individual." Dance/movement therapy effects changes in feelings, cognition, physical functioning, and behavior.

Dance as therapy came into existence in the 1940s, especially through the pioneering efforts of Marian Chace. Psychiatrists in Washington, D.C. found that their patients were deriving benefits from attending Chace's unique dance classes. As a result, Chace was asked to work on the back wards of St. Elizabeth's Hospital with patients who had been considered too disturbed to participate in regular group activities. A non-verbal group approach was needed and dance/movement therapy met that need.

The American Dance Therapy Association (ADTA) was founded in 1966 by 73 charter members in 15 states. Now, the Association has grown to nearly 1200 members in 46 states and 20 foreign countries. ADTA maintains a

About This Chapter: Information in this chapter is from "Dance/Movement Therapy." © 2005 American Dance Therapy Association. All rights reserved. Reprinted with permission. For additional information, visit http://www.adta.org.

registry of dance/movement therapists who meet specific educational and clinical practice standards. The title "Dance Therapist Registered" (DTR) is granted to entry-level dance/movement therapists who have a master's degree, which includes 700 hours of supervised clinical internship. The advanced level of registry, Academy of Dance Therapists Registered (ADTR), is awarded only after DTRs have completed 3,640 hours of supervised clinical work in an agency, institution, or special school, with additional supervision from an ADTR. In addition, as part of their written application for review by the credentials committee, applicants for ADTR must document their understanding of theory and practice.

The association has a code of ethics and has established standards for professional practice, education, and training. Dance/movement therapy academic programs stress coursework in dance/movement therapy theory and practice, movement observation and analysis, human development, psychopathology, cultural diversity, research skills, and group work. In 1979, ADTA established an approval process for the purpose of evaluating these programs. Research and scholarly writings are published in the *American Journal of Dance Therapy* and in publications funded by the Marian Chace Memorial Fund of the ADTA.

Today, in addition to those with severe emotional disorders, people of all ages and varying conditions receive dance/movement therapy. Examples of these are individuals with eating disorders, adult survivors of violence, sexually and physically abused children, dysfunctional families, the homeless, autistic children, the frail elderly, and substance abusers.

Research has been undertaken on the effects of dance/movement therapy in special settings (such as prisons and centers for the homeless) and with specific populations including the learning disabled,

> ♣ **It's A Fact!!**
>
> An evolving area of specialization is using dance/movement therapy in disease prevention and health promotion programs and with those who have chronic medical conditions. Many innovative programs provide dance/movement therapy for people with cardiovascular disease, hypertension, chronic pain, or breast cancer.

frail elderly, emotionally disturbed, depressed and suicidal, mentally retarded, substance abusers, visually and hearing impaired, psychotic, and autistic. Those with physical problems (such as amputations, traumatic brain injury, stroke, and chronic pain) and with chronic illnesses (such as anorexia and bulimia, cancer, Alzheimer's disease, cystic fibrosis, heart disease, diabetes, asthma, AIDS, and arthritis) have also been studied.

In institutions, dance/movement therapists may work as administrators as well as clinicians. Dance/movement therapists who are ADTRs in good standing are also qualified to teach, provide supervision, and engage in private practice.

Chapter 49

Humor Therapy

Definition Of Humor Therapy

Humor therapy is the art of using humor and laughter to help heal people with physical or mental illness.

Origins

The benefits of humor therapy were acknowledged as far back as the book of Proverbs in the Old Testament, which contains verses like Proverbs 17:22: "A cheerful heart is a good medicine, but a downcast spirit dries up the bones." The earliest historical reference to humor therapy is from the fourteenth century, when French surgeon Henri de Mondeville wrote, "Let the surgeon take care to regulate the whole regimen of the patient's life for joy and happiness, allowing his relatives and special friends to cheer him, and by having someone tell him jokes." In the sixteenth century, Martin Luther used a form of humor therapy as part of his pastoral counseling of depressed people. He advised them not to isolate themselves but to surround themselves with friends who could joke and make them laugh. Many of Luther's own letters to other people include playful or humorous remarks.

About This Chapter: Information in this chapter is from "Humor Therapy," from *Gale Encyclopedia Of Alternative Medicine*, by Ken R. Wells, 3 Thomson Gale, © 2005, Thomson/Gale. Reprinted by permission of The Gale Group.

Modern humor therapy dates from the 1930s, when clowns were brought into hospitals to cheer up children hospitalized with polio. In his 1979 book, *Anatomy of an Illness*, author Norman Cousins brought the subject of humor therapy to the attention of the medical community. Cousins, himself a physician, details how he used laughter to help ease his pain while undergoing treatment for rheumatoid arthritis of the spine (ankylosing spondylitis.) The benefits of laughter in treating the sick captured the public's attention in the 1998 movie *Patch Adams*, starring Robin Williams as real-life doctor Hunter "Patch" Adams. The movie is based on Adams' experiences treating the poor in rural West Virginia as related in his 1983 book *Gesundheit!*.

Benefits

It may seem difficult to measure the benefits of laughter in medicine, but a number of clinical studies have helped verify the adage that laughter is the best medicine.

Laughter appears to release tension in the diaphragm and relieve pressure on the liver and other internal organs. It stimulates the immune system, reduces stress, and helps balance the body's natural energy fields, or auras. People who have developed a strong sense of humor generally have a better sense of well-being and control in their lives.

✤ It's A Fact!!

Laughter improves the physical, mental, emotional, and spiritual health of individuals.

Source: *Gale Encyclopedia Of Alternative Medicine* © 2005.

A strong advocate of humor therapy is Dr. Michael R. Wasserman, president and chief medical officer of GeriMed Of America, Inc., a primary care physician management company for seniors. "A few years ago I came down with pneumonia, pulled out videotapes of *I Love Lucy* reruns and laughed myself back to good health," he said. "Clearly, humor and laughter have a positive effect on one's attitude and health overall. While we don't know all of the specifics, our immune system appears to benefit from these emotions."

Description

Humor therapy is used in both mainstream and alternative medicine. It can take many forms, but generally it is simply the recognition by physicians, nurses, and other health care practitioners of the value of mixing humor and laughter with medication and treatment. It is especially important with children and the elderly. Patients can also help themselves to heal by adding more humor and laughter to their lives.

Hospitals, hospices, nursing homes, and other medical care facilities can also turn to professionals for help in bringing humor to their patients. One example is the Big Apple Circus Clown Care Unit, which has programs in hospitals throughout the New York metropolitan area and major children's hospitals throughout the United States, including Children's Hospital in Boston. Professional clowns perform three days a week at the bedsides of hospitalized children to help ease the stress of serious illnesses. The clowns use juggling, mime, magic tricks, music, and gags to promote the healing power of humor. Instead of stethoscopes, thermometers, and hypodermics, the "doctors of delight" make their "clown rounds" with Groucho Marx disguises, funny hats, and rubber chickens.

Preparations

No advance preparation is required, except possibly a good repertoire of jokes and gags for the therapist.

Precautions

Not everyone will appreciate humor therapy. Some people may consider humor for the sick or injured as inappropriate or harmful. Therefore, it is important to know or sense when humor will be therapeutic and when it will be inappropriate. It should be used cautiously at first in situations in which the sensitivity of the person it is directed at is uncertain or unknown.

Side Effects

The only adverse side effects of humor therapy is that it can cause mental hurt, sadness, and alienation in persons who are not receptive to it, or if it is used insensitively.

Research And General Acceptance

Humor therapy is widely accepted in the alternative health community and is finding growing acceptance with mainstream health practitioners, especially registered nurses. Numerous scientific studies done in a clinical setting support the benefits of humor therapy. Two 1989 studies done at the Loma Linda (CA) University School of Medicine showed that laughter stimulates the immune system, counteracting the immunosuppressive effects of stress. These findings have been supported by other studies at the UCLA Medical School Department of Behavioral Medicine, Ohio State University School of Medicine, and the VA Medical Center in San Diego.

While several studies have demonstrated that humor therapy raises the level of salivary immunoglobin A, they have also been challenged. Other research focuses on the effects of humor therapy on natural killer (NK) cell assays, which are considered to give clearer and more replicable results. The general conclusion is that laughter has the potential to reduce stress and stress hormone levels, consequently reducing their effects on the immune system. Humor therapy may well be a useful complementary therapy for oncology patients.

Training And Certification

Although no official training or certification is required, there are a few institutions that teach humor therapy. Further information is available from the American Association for Applied and Therapeutic Humor.

American Association for Applied and Therapeutic Humor
Historic Mill Hill District
247 East Front Street
Trenton, NJ 08611
Phone: 609-392-0200
Fax: 609-392-0244
Website: http://www.aath.org

Chapter 50

Light Therapy

What is seasonal affective disorder (SAD)? Everyone gets "the winter blues"—what's different about SAD?

Many people complain of feeling down, having less energy, putting on a few pounds, and having difficulty getting up in the morning throughout the dark, short days of winter. People suffering from SAD experience these and other symptoms to such a degree that they feel unable to function normally. They often feel chronically depressed and fatigued, and want to withdraw from the world and to avoid social contacts. They become less productive at work and complain that their quality of life has gone. In the extreme, they may increase their sleep by as much as four hours or more per day, have greatly increased appetite, sometimes accompanied by irresistible cravings for sweet and starchy foods, and gain a substantial amount of weight. Women frequently report worsening of premenstrual symptoms.

An individual SAD sufferer, however, need not show all the symptoms described above. Sleep duration, for example, may be normal while carbohydrate craving may be extreme, or vice versa. Sometimes a symptom in the cluster is actually opposite the norm, such as insomnia as opposed to excessive

About This Chapter: "Questions and Answers about Seasonal Affective Disorder and Light Therapy," http://www.sltbr.org/sadfaq.htm. © 2000 Society for Light Treatment and Biological Rhythms. Reprinted with permission. Reviewed April 2006 by David A. Cooke, M.D., Diplomate, American Board of Internal Medicine.

sleep. A proper diagnosis of SAD requires a professional evaluation by a psychiatrist, psychologist or social worker. Although people with SAD often diagnose themselves correctly, professional confirmation is very important because certain medical conditions can be misdiagnosed as SAD, and because people can become depressed for many reasons aside from changes in their physical environment.

♣ **It's A Fact!!**

People with seasonal affective disorder (SAD) suffer in the extreme the kinds of changes that many others experience to a much lesser degree in wintertime.

Recent studies indicate that about three times as many people suffer from "winter doldrums," a sub-clinical level of SAD, as suffer at a level of clinical severity. These people notice the return of SAD-like symptoms each winter and are bothered by them, but remain fully functional.

What is light therapy for winter symptoms, and how is it delivered?

Light therapy involves exposure to intense light under specified conditions. The recommended light therapy system consists of a set of fluorescent bulbs installed in a box with a plastic diffusing screen and set up on a table or desk top at which one can sit comfortably for the treatment session. Treatment consists simply of sitting close to the light box with lights on and eyes open. Looking at the lights is not necessary or recommended; rather, one is free to engage in such activities as reading and writing or eating meals. What is important is to orient the head and body toward the lights, concentrating on activities on the surfaces illuminated by the lights, and not on the lights themselves. Treatment sessions can last from 15 minutes to 2 hours, usually once a day, but sometimes split into separate sessions, depending on individual needs and equipment used. The amount of light reaching the eyes and the duration of light treatments may need to be adjusted to achieve the best possible effect. It may be possible to shorten the duration of exposure by using a light source that gives off more light, or by sitting closer to the lights. It is important, however, to stay within the recommended guidelines that come with the lighting system.

Early research used special "full-spectrum" bulbs producing light similar in color composition to outdoor daylight, but more recent devices have used ordinary fluorescent bulbs (cool white, warm white, and triphosphor types) with similar results. (Since full-spectrum bulbs are designed to include ultraviolet light, which might contribute to cataract formation and skin problems, it is best to avoid such light at high intensity unless it has been carefully filtered for UV.) What appears to be critical is that the level of light produced match that of visible light outdoors shortly after sunrise or before sunset. Light intensity is critical for adequate therapy. Systems deliver varying amounts of light, which should be specified in detail by the manufacturer, with information provided as to how far away the patient should sit in order to receive the rated intensity.

Two recent innovations in apparatus design are worth noting. One is a head-mounted lighting unit that allows the user to move around while taking the treatment. Extensive testing of one such unit, however, was inconclusive. Although users reported feeling less depressed, it is not clear that this was more than a placebo effect. In principle, there is no reason why head-mounted units should not work effectively, provided that sufficient light gets to the eye. Further research and design enhancements may be needed to clarify the potential of this method.

A second type of innovation has been the design of dawn/dusk generators, which present graduated light signals in the bedroom as substitutes for (or as supplements to) bright light exposure. Although it is too soon to make a strong conclusion about clinical effectiveness because of the small number of studies, the use of simulated dawn signals appears to be antidepressant. Nonetheless, additional research is needed before a recommendation can be made.

♣ **It's A Fact!!**
As much as 25 percent of the population at the middle-to-northern latitudes of the United States experience "winter doldrums."

Is increased exposure to normal room light therapeutic, without the use of special apparatus?

For many people with winter depression, and especially those with the milder "doldrums," it can be helpful to increase the amount of indoor lighting with regular lamps. This is also true for people who live or work in dim environments. However, research studies show that most sufferers of SAD and winter doldrums require exposure to much higher light levels. Such therapeutic levels are usually at least five times higher (as measured in lux or foot-candles by a light meter) than provided by ordinary indoor lamps and ceiling fixtures in the home or office.

If outdoor light intensities are what's critical, can the therapeutic effect be achieved by spending more time outdoors in winter? Does this depend on the timing or the light?

Some people report improvement by spending more time outdoors where light intensity (even when it is overcast) can far exceed that of indoor light. For some, however, it appears that the strongest therapeutic effect requires exposure to artificial bright light in early morning at an hour (6:30 a.m., for example) when it is still quite dark outdoors during long winter nights. For others, however, the time of day of treatment doesn't seem to make a difference, and afternoon or evening light may also work. (Light taken very shortly before bedtime, however, may cause insomnia.) Those people who can sleep later on winter mornings may benefit by outdoor light exposure after awakening. Although just going outside may be adequate (weather permitting), looking directly at the sun must be avoided as it could cause eye damage.

Do the lights really work?

Researchers at medical centers and clinics in the U.S., Canada, Europe, Asia, and Australia have had much success with light therapy in many thousands of patients with clear histories of SAD for at least several years. Marked improvement is usually observed within four or five days, if not sooner, and symptoms

> ### ❖ It's A Fact!!
> The number of clinicians offering light therapy is increasing dramatically year by year, though compared to drug treatments or psychotherapy, the method is not yet in widespread use.

often return in about the same amount of time when the lights are withdrawn. Some people take longer than the usual few days to respond to light. It is therefore worth persevering for a week or two before concluding that light therapy doesn't work. Most users maintain a consistent daily schedule of light exposures beginning, as needed, in fall or winter and usually continuing until spring when outdoor light becomes sufficient to maintain good mood and high energy. Some people can skip treatments for one to three days, occasionally longer, without ill effect, but most start to slump quickly when treatment is interrupted.

How do the lights work?

The therapeutic level of illumination has several known physiological effects, though its mechanism of effect is still unclear. Blood levels of the hormone melatonin, which may be abnormally high at certain times of day, are rapidly reduced by light exposure. Depending on when bright light is presented, the body's internal clock, which controls daily rhythms of body temperature, hormone secretions, and sleep patterns, shifts ahead or is delayed when stimulated by light. These physiological time shifts may be the basis of the therapeutic response. On the other hand, the antidepressant effect may not involve rhythm shifts, but rather overall changes in neurotransmitter (chemicals involved in the communication between brain cells) activity. Neurotransmitters such as serotonin and dopamine may be prime candidates. Research into possible mechanisms is currently underway, and the final answer is not yet in.

Are there any side effects?

Side effects have been minimal. People occasionally report eye irritation and redness that can be alleviated by sitting farther from the lights or for shorter periods. Using a humidifier to counteract the dryness of winter air indoors may also help. A few people have reported feeling mildly nauseous or agitated when beginning light treatment; this tends to pass quickly as one accommodates to the high intensity. The most dramatic side effect, and one that occurs infrequently, is a switch from the lethargic state to an over-active state in which one may have difficulty getting a normal amount of sleep, become restless, even reckless, and be unable to slow down, feel irritable or subjectively speedy and "too high." This state is called hypomania, when milder, and mania when more severe. People who have previously experienced these states in late spring or summer are particularly vulnerable. In such cases, the guidance of a clinician skilled in the use of light therapy is important. For example, the dose of light should be reduced, and other treatments may be required.

Do the lights cause tanning?

They shouldn't. Most light therapy systems shield out the ultraviolet rays that causes tanning, or substantially reduce them, in order to avoid harmful effects of UV. Occasionally a person with sensitive skin shows reddening under full-spectrum lights, in which case complete UV blocking with filters, alternate bulbs or a sun screen lotion is needed. This should not influence effectiveness, however; the action of light therapy is through the eyes, not the skin, and in adults UV does not reach the retina (unfiltered artificial lens implants are an exception).

Can the lights be combined with antidepressant medication?

Patients who have received partial benefit from antidepressants often begin light therapy without changing drug dose. If there is quick improvement, it is then sometimes possible to withdraw the drugs (or reduce drug dose) under clinical supervision while maintaining improved mood and energy. Some patients find a combination of light and drug treatment to be most effective. Some antidepressant drugs (as well as lithium, St. John's Wort, and melatonin), however, are known or suspected to be "photo sensitizers," i.e., they may interact with the effect of light in the retina of the eyes. Users of antidepressant or other drugs should check with their physician or ophthalmologist (eye specialist) before commencing light treatment.

When should the lights not be used?

No adverse effects of light therapy have been found in ophthalmological (eye) examinations of SAD patients after treatment, but caution is warranted in people with pre-existing eye disease. There are several conditions (such as macular degeneration, retinitis pigmentosa, diabetic retinopathy) for which light therapy should be used only in conjunction with ophthalmological monitoring. Certain medications may increase the eye's sensitivity to light, and patients using them should also be followed by an ophthalmologist.

How did this treatment develop? How long has it been in use?

The first demonstration of clinical effect was in the early 1980s. Soon after, several research centers initiated clinical trials, and more than 2,500 SAD patients have been studied to date. The method has also been used in private practices, in most cases by psychiatrists, but also by family doctors, psychologists, and psychiatric social workers and nurses.

Are the lights medically approved? Is a prescription needed? Does insurance cover their cost?

The American Psychiatric Association, the U.S. Public Health Service Agency for Health Care Policy and Research, a Canadian Consensus Group of clinician-researchers, and the Society for Light Treatment and Biological Rhythms (SLTBR) have published clinical guidelines and endorsed the use of light treatment for winter depression. The light apparatus is not a prescription item, and its therapeutic use is currently still under consideration by the Food and Drug Administration (FDA). Pending FDA's decision in the matter, its authority cannot be superseded by guidelines that have been issued by other agencies. Light boxes are commercially available, but anyone suffering serious depression should seek a doctor's recommendation before obtaining a unit, and use it under the doctor's supervision. Some people have been successful in obtaining insurance reimbursement for purchase of light therapy apparatus, based on their physician's statement that the lights are medically indicated and effective for the individuals. Medicaid does not yet cover this expense.

The SLTBR makes available to clinicians a packet of information, including a statement of their position on light therapy for SAD, for use in supporting insurance claims. If the insurance policy covers psychiatric care or psychotherapy, it is very likely that it will reimburse for clinical sessions involved in diagnosis of SAD, evaluation for light treatment, and follow-up supervision.

How much do the lights cost? Can individuals build them for personal use?

Light therapy apparatus is available from several manufacturers at prices ranging from approximately $200 to $500, depending on how elaborate the design features are. Home construction of the apparatus is not recommended. Output must be specifically calibrated for the proper therapeutic effect. A danger of creating electrical or heat hazard also exists. The apparatus on the market should have been carefully evaluated for output intensity, compatibility of components, visual comfort, and maximum transmittance with minimal heat build-up and, importantly, clinical efficacy in controlled studies. These factors should be checked before purchasing any light system. Even though companies are not permitted to make medical claims for apparatus, some commercial devices do meet the standards of those that have been used in published research.

Is free treatment available?

Free treatment is available for research volunteers at SAD clinical research centers in the United States, Canada, Europe, Japan, Australia, and elsewhere. Recruitment for the winter season often begins in late summer or early fall.

> **✔ Quick Tip**
> The Society for Light Treatment and Biological Rhythms does not recommend that people with SAD treat themselves without the supervision of a qualified professional.

Can I treat my SAD symptoms on my own?

Like other forms of depression, SAD can seriously disrupt a person's functioning and quality of life. Light therapy needs to be monitored in order to achieve the best possible clinical outcome and fewest possible side effects. For some people, other therapies may be required in conjunction with lights. For these reasons, a knowledgeable professional is an invaluable resource in treating SAD.

What other treatments are available for SAD?

Apart from moving to or taking long vacations in a climate with more available natural light, some sufferers find that standard antidepressant medications provide a measure of relief, even if they do not reach their normal level of well-being until spring or summer. Although light therapy is often fully adequate for treating SAD, patients have been helped by other means as well, including psychotherapy, stress management, and exercise.

Is light treatment useful for conditions other than SAD?

Certain seasonal problems focused on winter can occur without depressed mood, such as increased appetite with overeating and weight gain, oversleeping, daytime fatigue, and worsening of premenstrual symptoms.

(Of course, these problems are often also associated with SAD). Light therapy has been used successfully in such cases, although additional research is still needed. Applications for certain non-seasonal problems also appear promising. One is for treatment of delayed sleep phase disorder, in which a person cannot fall asleep till very late nor awaken at any early-morning hour. The method may also be useful to assist with jet-lag adjustments, when a person's internal clock gets out of sync with local time because of rapid crossing over time zones. Shift workers may also benefit by appropriately timed bright light exposure to ease the adjustment to rotations as well as to counteract difficulties on the night shift. Light therapy may also be useful for non-seasonal depression, bulimia nervosa, and premenstrual syndrome.

Chapter 51

Music Therapy

What is music therapy?

Music therapy is an established healthcare profession that uses music to address physical, emotional, cognitive, and social needs of individuals of all ages. Music therapy improves the quality of life for persons who are well and meets the needs of children and adults with disabilities or illnesses. Music therapy interventions can be designed to do the following:

- Promote wellness
- Alleviate pain
- Enhance memory
- Promote physical rehabilitation

- Manage stress
- Express feelings
- Improve communication

What do music therapists do?

Music therapists assess emotional well-being, physical health, social functioning, communication abilities, and cognitive skills through musical responses; design music sessions for individuals and groups based on client needs using music improvisation, receptive music listening, song writing, lyric discussion, music and imagery, music performance, and learning through music; participate in interdisciplinary treatment planning, ongoing evaluation, and follow up.

Who can benefit from music therapy?

Children, adolescents, adults, and the elderly with mental health needs, developmental and learning disabilities, Alzheimer's disease, and other aging related conditions, substance abuse problems, brain injuries, physical disabilities, and acute and chronic pain, including mothers in labor.

> ♣ **It's A Fact!!**
> Research in music therapy supports its effectiveness in a wide variety of healthcare and educational settings.
>
> Source: "Music Therapy Makes a Difference." © American Music Therapy Association.

Where do music therapists work?

Music therapists work in psychiatric hospitals, rehabilitative facilities, medical hospitals, outpatient clinics, day care treatment centers, agencies serving developmentally disabled persons, community mental health centers, drug and alcohol programs, senior centers, nursing homes, hospice programs, correctional facilities, halfway houses, schools, and private practice.

What is the history of music therapy as a health care profession?

The idea of music as a healing influence which could affect health and behavior is as least as old as the writings of Aristotle and Plato. The 20th century discipline began after World War I and World War II when community musicians of all types, both amateur and professional, went to veterans hospitals around the country to play for the thousands of veterans suffering both physical and emotional trauma from the wars. The patients' notable physical and emotional responses to music led the doctors and nurses to request the hiring of musicians by the hospitals. It was soon evident that the hospital musicians needed some prior training before entering the facility, and so the demand grew for a college curriculum. The first music therapy degree program in the world, founded at Michigan State University in 1944, celebrated its 50th anniversary in 1994. The American Music Therapy Association (AMTA) was founded in 1998 as a union of the National Association for Music Therapy and the American Association for Music therapy.

Who is qualified to practice music therapy?

Persons who complete one of the approved college music therapy curricula (including an internship) are then eligible to sit for the national examination offered by the Certification Board for Music Therapists. Music therapists who successfully complete the independently administered examination hold the music therapist-board certified credential (MT-BC).

The National Music Therapy Registry (NMTR) serves qualified music therapy professionals with the following designations: RMT, CMT, ACMT. These individuals have met accepted educational and clinical training standards and are qualified to practice music therapy.

Is there research to support music therapy?

AMTA promotes a vast amount of research exploring the benefits of music as therapy through publication of the *Journal of Music Therapy, Music Therapy Perspectives*, and other sources. A substantial body of literature exists to support the effectiveness of music therapy.

What are some misconceptions about music therapy?

That the client or patient has to have some particular music ability to benefit from music therapy—they do not. That there is one particular style of music that is more therapeutic than all the rest—this is not the case. All styles of music can be useful in effecting change in a client or patient's life. The individual's preferences, circumstances and need for treatment, and the client or patient's goals help to determine the types of music a music therapist may use.

How can healthy individuals apply music therapy techniques?

Healthy individuals can use music for stress reduction via active music making, such as drumming, as well as passive listening for relaxation. Music is often a vital support for physical exercise. Music therapy assisted labor and delivery may also be included in this category since pregnancy is regarded as a normal part of women's life cycles.

How is music therapy utilized in hospitals?

Music is used in general hospitals to: alleviate pain in conjunction with anesthesia or pain medication; elevate patients' mood and counteract depression; promote movement for physical rehabilitation; calm or sedate, often to induce sleep; counteract apprehension or fear; and lesson muscle tension for the purpose of relaxation, including the autonomic nervous system.

How is music therapy utilized in nursing homes?

Music is used with elderly persons to increase or maintain their level of physical, mental, and social/emotional functioning. The sensory and intellectual stimulation of music can help maintain a person's quality of life.

How is music therapy utilized in schools?

Music therapists are often hired in schools to provide music therapy services listed on the Individualized Education Plan for mainstreamed special learners. Music learning is used to strengthen nonmusical areas such as communication skills and physical coordination skills, which are important for daily life.

How is music therapy utilized in psychiatric facilities?

Music therapy allows persons with mental health needs to: explore personal feelings, make positive changes in mood and emotional states, have a sense of control over life through successful experiences, practice problem solving, and resolve conflicts leading to stronger family and peer relationships.

What is a typical music therapy session like?

Since music therapists serve a wide variety of persons with many different types of needs, there is no such thing as an overall typical session. Sessions are designed, and music selected, based on the individual client's treatment plan.

What is the future of music therapy?

The future of music therapy is promising. State-of-the-art music therapy research in physical rehabilitation, Alzheimer's disease, and psychoneuroimmunology is documenting the effectiveness of music therapy in terms that are important in the context of a biological medical model.

Part Eight

Alternative Treatments For Specific Diseases And Conditions

Chapter 52

Pain Management Using Complementary And Alternative Methods

Pain Treatments

In addition to medication, there are several techniques that can be useful in managing pain. These techniques can be used in conjunction with medication or, in some cases, can be used alone to effectively manage pain. Several alternative methods of pain control for cancer pain have been sanctioned by the National Institutes of Health sponsored jointly by the Office of Alternative Medicine and the Office of Medical Applications of Research. These include cognitive/behavioral techniques such as relaxation, distraction, and visualization and mind/body techniques such as hypnosis and biofeedback. Although there is limited scientific data to support some of these methods, the risks associated with using them are minimal. Moreover, many of these methods can be used any place or any time and some of them do not cost anything. Therefore, many of these techniques are worth trying because they might help give you more control of your pain.

About This Chapter: Information in this chapter under the heading "Pain Treatments" is from "Cancer Pain Treatments: Alternative/Complementary Methods." © 2000 Association of Cancer Online Resources. Reprinted with permission. Text under the heading "Questions and Answers About Using Magnets To Treat Pain" is from the National Center for Complementary and Alternative Medicine (NCCAM), National Institutes of Health, NCCAM Publication No. D208, May 2004. All of the text in this chapter was reviewed and updated June 2006 by David A. Cooke, M.D., Diplomate, American Board of Internal Medicine.

Cognitive/behavioral techniques such as relaxation, distraction, and visualization have been shown to reduce and control pain. Relaxation relieves pain or keeps it from getting worse by reducing tension in the muscles. It can help you fall asleep, give you more energy, make you less tired, reduce your anxiety, and make other pain relief methods work better. Relaxation can include quiet breathing, deep breathing, or progressive relaxation. Progressive relaxation is a technique used to reduce cancer pain in specific areas of the body. This technique entails lying down and successively clenching and releasing individual muscle groups, eventually focusing on those involved with the pain.

Distraction (that is, focusing your attention on something else) can be a powerful way of temporarily relieving even the most intense pain. Patients report that when concentrating on something else—music, television, talking to family or friends—pain is diminished. This can work especially well while waiting for pain medications to take effect. The use of a portable radio or CD player (with earphones) during painful procedures is especially helpful for some people.

Visualization involves the use of a personal symbol to imagine the transformation of pain; for example, you might imagine the pain as a red-hot fire and then visualize the pain diminishing as the fire is put out by water. Audiotapes are widely available to teach imagery and visualization skills. Meditation, in which a person focuses on his or her own breathing or the repetition of a word, phrase, or prayer, is another useful cognitive/behavioral method.

Physiatric techniques include a variety of methods including electrical stimulation (such as PENS and TENS), skin stimulation, therapeutic exercise, and the use of orthoses and assistive devices. Percutaneous electrical nerve stimulation (PENS) combines acupuncture with electrical stimulation of the nerves to achieve pain control. Transcutaneous electrical nerve stimulation (TENS) relieves pain by sending small electrical impulses through electrodes placed on the skin to underlying nerve fibers. Skin stimulation is the use of pressure, friction, temperature change, or chemical substances such as menthol to excite the nerve endings in the skin. When the skin is stimulated so that pressure, warmth, or cold is felt, the pain sensation is lessened or blocked. Therapeutic exercise, even exercise as minimal as range-of-motion exercise, can improve function and lessen pain. A physical therapist can prescribe an exercise program that may include stretching, strengthening, and conditioning. Several devices are available that may improve function and relieve pain such as wraps, pressure stockings, or pneumatic pump devices. Orthotic devices can immobilize and support painful or weakened areas of the body. Examples of orthotic devices include a splint on a painful limb or a collar for patients with neck or back pain.

Massage is another technique that can be very useful in managing pain. Massage increases blood circulation and relieves tension. Massage can be performed by anyone, from a trained massage therapist to a caregiver who is willing to give a simple massage. There are several devices on the market that enable you to add vibration and/or heat to a massage. One of the most gratifying aspects of massage is the simple fact that it involves one person touching and caring for another person.

Biofeedback techniques, which use special machines to help patients learn how to control certain body functions such as heart rate, blood pressure, and muscle tension, can help you reduce anxiety and help you cope with your pain. Personal, portable biofeedback equipment is available for home use.

Hypnosis can change how you perceive pain and reduce your anxiety. Under hypnosis, a patient enters a state of deep relaxation and then is given simple suggestions to experience the pain in a different way. Several studies have supported the effectiveness of hypnosis and imagery; hypnosis is effective in reducing dependence on opioids during bone marrow transplant procedures, and imagery is effective in providing pain relief from mucositis. Audiotapes for self-hypnosis are widely available for home use.

Other less common alternative/complementary methods include Chinese medicine, nutrition, and herbal remedies. Many cancer patients have used traditional Chinese medicine as an adjunct to conventional medical treatment. The use of acupuncture, with or without moxibustion (the burning of herbs at specific points over the skin), the ingestion of specific herbal patent remedies, and physical exercise programs such as qigong or tai chi have all been reported by patients to help control cancer pain. However, there has been little scientific study to determine whether these techniques are actually helpful.

Anecdotal information supports the use of nutrition and herbs to control pain indirectly. Herbs are mainly used to support immune functioning, promote the health of the liver, and detoxify the lymph system, with pain reduction being a secondary effect. Yerba mate tea has been found to decrease neuropathic pain associated with chemotherapy, and *Valeriana officinalis* is known to reduce pain and promote rest and sleep. If you are considering using nutrition or herbs to manage your pain, you should always consult a competent, well-trained practitioner before taking any nutritional or herbal supplements. Additionally, it is important that all your physicians are aware of any and all alternative treatments you may be doing. Many herbal preparations have significant interactions with prescription medication, some of which can be life threatening.

The lack of controlled outcome studies and the placebo effect (that is, just taking anything can make you feel better) influence the reliability of reports of the success of these treatments. You should always communicate with your doctor about alternative methods you are considering. The safety of most alternative methods has not been well assessed, and your medical provider may be able to advise you whether a given approach is likely to be harmful. If you have a strong desire to incorporate non-traditional alternative/complementary approaches into your care and your doctor is unreceptive to these approaches, you may want to find another doctor.

Questions And Answers About Using Magnets To Treat Pain

What are magnets?

Magnets are objects that produce a type of energy called magnetic fields. All magnets possess a property called polarity—that is, a magnet's power of attraction is strongest at its opposite ends,

♣ **It's A Fact!!**
Alternative and complementary approaches to pain management are dependent on the active participation by the patient and a close working relationship between the patient and the alternative practitioner (for example, the stress reduction counselor, the herbalist, the Chinese doctor, the acupuncturist).

Source: © 2000 Association of Cancer Online Resources.

usually called the north and south poles. The north and south poles attract each other, but north repels north and south repels south. All magnets attract iron.

Magnets come in different strengths, most often measured in units called gauss (G). For comparison purposes, the Earth has a magnetic field of about 0.5 G; refrigerator magnets range from 35 to 200 G; magnets marketed for the treatment of pain are usually 300 to 5,000 G; and MRI (magnetic resonance imaging) machines widely used to diagnose medical conditions non-invasively produce up to 200,000 G.

The vast majority of magnets marketed to consumers for health purposes are of a type called static (or permanent) magnets. They have magnetic fields that do not change.

The other magnets used for health purposes are called electromagnets because they generate magnetic fields only when electrical current flows through them. Passing an electric current through a wire coil wrapped around a magnetic core creates the magnetic field. Electromagnets can be pulsed— that is, the magnetic field is turned on and off very rapidly.

Is the use of magnets considered conventional medicine or complementary and alternative medicine?

There are some uses of electromagnets within conventional medicine. For example, scientists have found that electromagnets can be used to speed the healing of bone fractures that are not healing well. Even more commonly, electromagnets are used to map areas of the brain. However, most uses of magnets by consumers in attempts to treat pain are considered CAM because they have not been scientifically proven and are not part of the practice of conventional medicine.

What is the history of the discovery and use of magnets to treat pain?

Magnets have been used for many centuries in attempts to treat pain. By various accounts, this use began when people first noticed the presence of naturally magnetized stones, also called lodestones. Other accounts trace the beginning to a shepherd noticing that some stones pulled out the nails in his sandals. By the third century A.D., Greek physicians were using rings made of magnetized metal to treat arthritis and pills made of magnetized amber to stop bleeding. In the Middle Ages, doctors used magnets to treat gout, arthritis, poisoning, and baldness to probe and clean wounds and to retrieve arrowheads and other iron-containing objects from the body.

> ❦ **It's A Fact!!**
>
> Magnets have been marketed for a wide range of diseases and conditions, including pain, respiratory problems, high blood pressure, circulatory problems, arthritis, rheumatism, and stress. However, evidence of effectiveness is generally lacking.
>
> Source: National Center for Complementary and Alternative Medicine

In the United States, magnetic devices (such as hairbrushes and insoles), magnetic salves, and clothes with magnets applied came into wide use after the Civil War, especially in some rural areas where few doctors were available. Healers claimed that magnetic fields existed in the blood, organs, or elsewhere in the body and that people became ill when their magnetic fields were depleted. Thus, healers marketed magnets as a means of restoring these magnetic fields. Magnets were promoted as cures for paralysis, asthma, seizures, blindness, cancer, and other conditions. The use of magnets to treat medical problems remained popular well into the 20th century.

How common is the use of magnets to treat pain?

A 1999 survey of patients who had rheumatoid arthritis, osteoarthritis, or fibromyalgia, and who were seen by rheumatologists, reported that 18 percent had used magnets or copper bracelets, and that this was the second-most-used CAM therapy by these patients after chiropractic. One estimate places Americans' spending on magnets to treat pain at $500 million per year; the worldwide estimate is $5 billion. Many people purchase magnets in stores or over the internet to use on their own without consulting a health care provider.

What are some examples of theories and beliefs about magnets and pain?

Some examples of theories and beliefs about using magnets to treat pain are listed below. These range from theories proposed by scientific researchers to claims made by magnet manufacturers. It is important to note that while the results for some of the findings from the scientific studies have been intriguing, none of the theories or claims below has been conclusively proven.

- Static magnets might change how cells function.

- Magnets might alter or restore the equilibrium (balance) between cell death and growth.

- Because it contains iron, blood might act as a conductor of magnetic energy. Static magnets might increase the flow of blood and, therefore, increase the delivery of oxygen and nutrients to tissues.

- Weak pulsed electromagnets might affect how nerve cells respond to pain.

- Pulsed electromagnets might change the brain's perception of pain.

- Electromagnets might affect the production of white blood cells involved in fighting infection and inflammation.

- Magnets might increase the temperature of the area of the body being treated.

- Magnetizing or re-magnetizing drinking water or other beverages might allow them to hydrate the body better and flush out more toxins than ordinary drinking water.

How are static magnets used in attempts to treat pain?

Static magnets are usually made from iron, steel, rare-earth elements, or alloys. Typically, the magnets are placed directly on the skin or placed inside clothing or other materials that come into close contact with the body. Static magnets can be unipolar (one pole of the magnet faces or touches the skin) or bipolar (both poles face or touch the skin, sometimes in repeating patterns). Some magnet manufacturers make claims about the poles of magnets—for example, that a unipolar design is better than a bipolar design, or that the North Pole gives a different effect from the South Pole. These claims have not been scientifically proven.

How are electromagnets used in attempts to treat pain?

The FDA approved electromagnets in 1979 to treat bone fractures that have not healed well. Researchers have been studying electromagnets for painful conditions, such as knee pain from osteoarthritis, chronic pelvic pain, problems in bones and muscles, and migraine headaches. However, these uses of electromagnets are still considered experimental by the FDA and have not been approved. Currently, electromagnets to treat pain are being used mainly under the supervision of a health care provider and/or in clinical trials.

An electromagnetic therapy called TMS (transcranial magnetic stimulation) is also being studied by researchers. In TMS, an insulated coil is placed against the head, near the area of the brain to be examined or treated, and an electrical current generates a magnetic field into the brain. Currently, TMS is most often used as a diagnostic tool, but research is also under way to see whether it is effective in relieving pain. A type of TMS called rTMS (repetitive TMS) is believed by some to produce longer lasting effects and is being explored for its usefulness in treating chronic pain, facial pain, headache, and fibromyalgia pain. A related form of electromagnetic therapy is rMS (repetitive magnetic stimulation). It is similar to rTMS except that the magnetic coil is placed on or near a painful area of the body other than the head. This therapy is being studied as a treatment for musculoskeletal pain.

There have been a number of studies performed to study whether magnets are effective for various types of pain. Unfortunately, most of these studies have been small, and there have been conflicting results regarding whether they have any effect beyond placebos.

Are there scientific controversies associated with using magnets for pain?

Yes, there are many controversies. Examples include the following:

• The mechanism(s) by which magnets might relieve pain have not been conclusively identified or proven.

• Pain relief while using a magnet may be due to reasons other than the magnet. For example, there could be a placebo effect or the relief could come from whatever holds the magnet in place, such as a warm bandage or a cushioned insole.

• Opinions differ among manufacturers, health care providers who use magnetic therapy, and others about which types of magnets (strength, polarity, length of use, and other factors) should be used and how they should be used in studies to give the most definitive answers.

• Actual magnet strengths can vary (sometimes widely) from the strengths claimed by manufacturers. This can affect scientists' ability to reproduce the findings of other scientists and consumers' ability to know what strength magnet they are actually using.

Despite some positive reports, magnets have never been consistently proven effective for pain treatment, and a number of studies have failed to find any effect.

Have any side effects or complications occurred from using magnets for pain?

The kinds of magnets marketed to consumers are generally considered to be safe when applied to the skin. Reports of side effects or complications have been rare. One study reported that a small percentage of participants had bruising or redness on their skin where a magnet was worn.

Manufacturers often recommend that the following people not use static magnets:

• Pregnant women, because the possible effects of magnets on the fetus are not known

- People who use a medical device such as a pacemaker, defibrillator, or insulin pump, because magnets may affect the magnetically controlled features of such devices

- People who use a patch that delivers medication through the skin, in case magnets cause dilation of blood vessels, which could affect the delivery of the medicine. This caution also applies to people with an acute sprain, inflammation, infection, or wound.

There have been rare cases of problems reported from the use of electromagnets. Because at present these are being used mainly under the supervision of a health care provider and/or in clinical trials, readers are advised to consult their provider about any questions.

What should consumers know if they are considering using magnets to treat pain?

- It is important that people inform all their health care providers about any therapy they are using or considering, including magnetic therapy. This is to help ensure a safe and coordinated plan of care.

- In the studies that did find benefits from magnetic therapy, many have shown those benefits very quickly. This suggests that if a magnet does work, it should not take very long for the user to start noticing the effect. Therefore, people may wish to purchase

---

✔ Quick Tip
Tips On Buying A Magnet

The U.S. Food and Drug Administration and the Pennsylvania Medical Society suggest the following:

- Check on the company's reputation with consumer protection agencies.

- Watch for high return fees. If you see them before purchase, ask that they be dropped and obtain written confirmation that they will be.

- Pay by credit card if possible. This offers you more protection if there is a problem.

- If you buy from sources (such as websites) that are not based in the United States, U.S. law can do little to protect you if you have a problem related to the purchase.

Source: National Center for Complementary and Alternative Medicine.

magnets with a 30-day return policy and return the product if they do not get satisfactory results within 1 to 2 weeks.

• If people decide to use magnets and they experience side effects that concern them, they should stop using the magnets and contact their health care providers.

• Consumers who are considering magnets, whether for pain or other conditions, can consult the free publications prepared by federal government agencies.

Is the National Center for Complementary and Alternative Medicine (NCCAM) funding research on magnets for pain and other diseases and conditions?

Yes. For example, recent projects supported by NCCAM include the following:

• Static magnets for fibromyalgia pain and quality of life

• Pulsed electromagnets for migraine headache pain

• Static magnets for their effects on networks of blood vessels involved in healing

• TMS for Parkinson's disease

• Electromagnets for their effects on injured nerve and muscle cells

Chapter 53

Cancer And Complementary And Alternative Medicine

Questions And Answers About Cancer And Complementary And Alternative Medicine

Is complementary and alternative medicine (CAM) widely used by cancer patients?

According to the most recent comprehensive survey on Americans' use of CAM, 36 percent of U.S. adults are using some form of CAM. When megavitamin therapy and prayer for health reasons are included in the definition of CAM, that percentage rises to 62 percent. These results are based on the 2002 National Health Interview Survey, which was supported by the National Center for Complementary and Alternative Medicine (NCCAM)

About This Chapter: This chapter begins with "Questions And Answers About Cancer And Complementary And Alternative Medicine," excerpted from "Cancer and Complementary and Alternative Medicine," National Center for Complementary and Alternative Medicine (NCCAM), National Institutes of Health, NCCAM Publication No. D286, September 2005. Text under the heading "Acupuncture As A Cancer Treatment," is excerpted from PDQ® Cancer Information Summary. National Cancer Institute; Bethesda, MD. "Acupuncture (PDQ®): Complementary and Alternative Medicine - Patient," Updated 05/2006. Accessed 06/07/2006. Text under the heading "Spirituality In Cancer Care," is excerpted from PDQ® Cancer Information Summary. National Cancer Institute; Bethesda, MD. "Spirituality in Cancer Care (PDQ®) - Patient," Updated 01/2006. Accessed 06/07/2006.

and the National Center for Health Statistics (part of the Centers for Disease Control and Prevention). The survey found that rates of CAM use are especially high among patients with serious illnesses such as cancer.

Several smaller studies of CAM use by cancer patients have been conducted. A study of CAM use in patients with cancer in the July 2000 issue of the *Journal of Clinical Oncology* found that 69 percent of 453 cancer patients had used at least one CAM therapy as part of their cancer treatment. A study published in the December 2004 issue of the *Journal of Clinical Oncology* reported that 88 percent of 102 people with cancer who were enrolled in phase I clinical trials (research studies in people) at the Mayo Comprehensive Cancer Center had used at least one CAM therapy. Of those, 93 percent had used supplements (such as vitamins or minerals), 53 percent had used non-supplement forms of CAM (such as prayer/spiritual practices or chiropractic care), and almost 47 percent had used both.

A review article in the March 2005 issue of the *Southern Medical Journal* reported that cancer patients take supplements to reduce side effects and organ toxicity, to protect and stimulate their immune systems, or to prevent further cancers or recurrences. Patients frequently see using supplements as a way to take control over their health and increase their quality of life.

How are CAM approaches evaluated?

The same rigorous scientific evaluation used to assess conventional cancer treatments should be used for CAM therapies. NCCAM is funding a number of clinical trials to evaluate CAM therapies for cancer.

Conventional cancer treatments are studied for safety and effectiveness through a rigorous scientific process that includes laboratory research and clinical trials with large numbers of patients. Less is known about the safety and effectiveness of complementary and alternative methods to treat cancer, although some CAM therapies have undergone rigorous evaluation.

A small number of CAM therapies, which were originally considered to be purely alternative approaches, are finding a place in cancer treatment—not as cures, but as complementary therapies that may help patients feel better and recover faster. One example is acupuncture. In 1997, a panel of

---

✤ It's A Fact!!

The National Center for Complementary and Alternative Medicine (NCCAM) is sponsoring a number of clinical trials (research studies in people) to study complementary and alternative medicine (CAM) therapies for cancer. (Source: NCCAM)

---

experts at the National Institutes of Health (NIH) Consensus Conference found acupuncture to be effective in managing chemotherapy-associated nausea and vomiting and in controlling pain associated with surgery. In contrast, some approaches, such as the use of laetrile, have been studied and found ineffective or potentially harmful.

Is NCCAM sponsoring clinical trials on CAM for cancer?

NCCAM is sponsoring a number of clinical trials to study complementary and alternative treatments for cancer. Some of these trials study the effects of complementary approaches used in addition to conventional treatments, while others compare alternative therapies with conventional treatments. Recent trials include the following:

- Acupuncture to relieve neck and shoulder pain following surgery for head or neck cancer

- Ginger as a treatment for nausea and vomiting caused by chemotherapy

- Massage for the treatment of cancer pain

- Mistletoe extract combined with chemotherapy for the treatment of solid tumors

Patients who are interested in taking part in these or any other clinical trials should talk with their health care provider.

What should cancer patients do when using or considering CAM therapies?

Cancer patients who are using or considering CAM should discuss this decision with their health care provider, as they would any therapy. Some complementary and alternative therapies may interfere with standard treatment or may be harmful when used along with standard treatment.

As with any medicine or treatment, it is a good idea to learn about the therapy, including whether the results of scientific studies support the claims that are made for it.

When considering CAM, what questions should cancer patients ask their health care providers?

- What benefits can be expected from this therapy?

- What are the risks associated with this therapy?

- Do the known benefits outweigh the risks?

- What are the potential side effects?

- Will the therapy interfere with conventional treatment?

- Is this therapy part of a clinical trial? If so, who is sponsoring the trial?

- Will the therapy be covered by health insurance?

Acupuncture As A Cancer Treatment

Scientific studies on the use of acupuncture to treat cancer and side effects of cancer began only recently. Laboratory and animal studies suggest that acupuncture can reduce nausea caused by chemotherapy and may help the immune system be stronger during chemotherapy.

Most studies of the use of acupuncture in cancer patients have been done in China. In 197, the National Institutes of Health (NIH) began evaluating the safety and effectiveness of acupuncture as a complementary and alternative therapy.

- **Studies of the effect of acupuncture on the immune system.** Human studies on the effect of acupuncture on the immune system of cancer patients showed that it improved immune system response.

- **Studies of the effect of acupuncture on pain.** In clinical studies, acupuncture reduced the amount of pain in some cancer patients. In one study, most of the patients treated with acupuncture were able to stop taking drugs for pain relief or to take smaller doses. The findings from these studies are not considered strong, however, because of weaknesses in study design and size. Studies using strict scientific methods are needed to prove how acupuncture affects pain.

• **Studies of the effect of acupuncture on nausea and vomiting caused by chemotherapy.** The strongest evidence of the effect of acupuncture has come from clinical trials on the use of acupuncture to relieve nausea and vomiting. Several types of clinical trials using different acupuncture methods showed acupuncture reduced nausea and vomiting caused by chemotherapy, surgery, and morning sickness.

• **Studies of the effect of acupuncture on cancer and symptoms (other than nausea) caused by cancer treatment.** Clinical trials are studying the effects of acupuncture on cancer and symptoms caused by cancer treatment, including weight loss, cough, chest pain, fever, anxiety, depression, night sweats, hot flashes, dry mouth, speech problems, and fluid in the arms or legs. Studies have shown that, for many patients, treatment with acupuncture either relieves symptoms or keeps them from getting worse.

There have been few complications reported. Problems are caused by using needles that are not sterile (free of germs) and from placing the needle in the wrong place, movement of the patient, or a defect in the needle. Problems include soreness and pain during treatment, feeling tired, lightheaded, or sleepy, and infections. Because chemotherapy and radiation therapy weaken the body's immune system, a strict clean needle method must be used when acupuncture treatment is given to cancer patients. It is important to seek treatment from a qualified acupuncture practitioner who uses a new set of disposable (single-use) needles for each patient.

Spirituality In Cancer Care

Many cancer patients rely on spiritual and/or religious beliefs and practices to help them cope with their disease. This is called spiritual coping. Some patients may want their doctors and caregivers to address spiritual concerns, not only for end-of-life issues but also during treatment. Medical staff may therefore ask patients to identify spiritual issues that are important to them during cancer care.

Definition Of Spirituality And Religion

For many people, spirituality and religion have different meanings. The terms spirituality and religion are often used in place of each other, but for many people they have different meanings. Religion may be defined as a specific set of beliefs and practices, usually associated with an organized group. Spirituality may be defined as an individual's sense of peace, purpose, and connection to others, and beliefs about the meaning of life. Spirituality may be found and expressed through an organized religion or in other ways. Many patients consider themselves both spiritual and religious. Some patients may consider themselves spiritual, but not religious. Other patients may consider themselves religious, but not spiritual.

Spiritual distress is unresolved religious or spiritual conflict and doubt. A serious illness like cancer may challenge a patient's beliefs or religious values, resulting in high levels of spiritual distress. Some cancer patients may feel that cancer is a punishment by God or may suffer a loss of faith after being diagnosed.

Other patients may experience mild spiritual distress when coping with cancer. For example, when prayer is used as a coping method, some patients may worry about how to pray or may doubt their prayers are being answered.

Relation Of Spirituality To Quality Of Life

Spiritual and religious well-being may be associated with improved quality of life. It is not known for sure how spirituality is related to health. Some research shows that spiritual or religious beliefs and practices promote a positive mental attitude that may help a patient feel better. Spiritual and religious well-being may be associated with improved quality of life in the following ways:

• Reduced anxiety, depression, and discomfort

• Reduced sense of isolation (feeling alone)

• Better adjustment to the effects of cancer and its treatment

• Increased ability to enjoy life during cancer treatment

• A feeling of personal growth as a result of living with cancer

• Improved health outcomes

Spiritual distress may contribute to poorer health outcomes. High levels of spiritual distress may interfere with the patient's ability to cope with cancer and cancer treatment. This distress may contribute to poorer health outcomes and less satisfaction with life. Health care providers may encourage patients to seek advice from appropriate spiritual or religious leaders to help resolve their conflicts, which may improve their health, quality of life, and ability to cope.

Screening And Assessment

A spiritual assessment may help the doctor understand if a patient will use religious or spiritual beliefs to cope with the cancer diagnosis and treatment. Knowing the role that religion and spirituality play in the patient's life may help the doctor understand how religious and spiritual beliefs affect the patient's response to the cancer diagnosis and decisions about cancer treatment. Some doctors or caregivers may wait for the patient to bring up spiritual concerns. Others will ask for some initial information in an interview or on a form called a spiritual assessment.

A spiritual assessment will include asking about religious preference, beliefs, and spiritual practices. Medical staff may not ask about every issue the patient feels is important. The patient should feel comfortable bringing up other spiritual or religious issues that he or she thinks may affect cancer care.

A spiritual assessment may include questions relating to the following issues:

- Religious denomination, if any
- Beliefs or philosophy of life
- Important spiritual practices or rituals
- Use of spirituality or religion as a source of strength
- Participation in a religious community
- Use of prayer or meditation
- Loss of faith
- Conflicts between spiritual or religious beliefs and cancer treatments

- Ways the caregivers may address the patient's spiritual needs

- Concerns about death and the afterlife

- End-of-life planning

Meeting The Patient's Spiritual And Religious Needs

In addressing a patient's spiritual needs during cancer care, medical staff will take their lead from the wishes of the patient. Spirituality and religion are very personal decisions. Patients can expect doctors and caregivers to respect their religious and spiritual beliefs and concerns. A cancer patient who relies on spirituality to cope with the disease may count on medical staff to respect that practice with support and referrals to appropriate spiritual or religious resources. Patients who do not choose to have spiritual issues addressed during cancer care may also count on medical staff to respect and support their views.

Doctors and caregivers will try to respond to their patients' concerns, but may avoid taking part in patients' religious rituals or debating religious beliefs.

Doctors may address a patient's spiritual needs in setting goals and planning treatment. Doctors may address a patient's spiritual needs in the following ways:

- Identifying goals for care and making medical decisions that are consistent with the patient's spiritual and/or religious views and which also enable the doctor to maintain the integrity of his or her own spiritual and/or religious views.

- Respectfully supporting the patient's use of spiritual coping during the illness.

- Encouraging patients to speak with their clergy or spiritual leader.

- Referring the patient to a hospital chaplain, appropriate religious leader, or support group that addresses spiritual issues during illness.

Chapter 54

Diabetes And Complementary And Alternative Medicine

Some people with diabetes use complementary or alternative therapies to treat diabetes. Although some of these therapies may be effective, others can be ineffective or even harmful. Patients who use complementary and alternative medicine need to let their health care providers know what they are doing.

Some complementary and alternative medicine therapies are discussed in this chapter. For more information, talk with your health care provider.

Acupuncture

Acupuncture is a procedure in which a practitioner inserts needles into designated points on the skin. Some scientists believe that acupuncture triggers the release of the body's natural painkillers. Acupuncture has been shown to offer relief from chronic pain. People with neuropathy, the painful nerve damage of diabetes, sometimes use acupuncture.

About This Chapter: Information in this chapter is from "Complementary and Alternative Medical Therapies for Diabetes," National Diabetes Information Clearinghouse (NDIC), a service of the National Institute of Diabetes and Digestive and Kidney Diseases (NIDDK), National Institutes of Health (NIH), NIH Publication No. 04-4552, May 2004.

Biofeedback

Biofeedback is a technique that helps a person become more aware of and learn to deal with the body's response to pain. This alternative therapy emphasizes relaxation and stress-reduction techniques. Guided imagery is a relaxation technique that some professionals who use biofeedback do. With guided imagery, a person thinks of peaceful mental images, such as ocean waves. A person may also include the images of controlling or curing a chronic disease, such as diabetes. People using this technique believe their condition can be eased with these positive images.

Chromium

The benefit of added chromium for diabetes has been studied and debated for several years. Several studies report that chromium supplementation may improve diabetes control. Chromium is needed to make glucose tolerance factor, which helps insulin improve its action. Because of insufficient information on the use of chromium to treat diabetes, no recommendations for supplementation yet exist.

Ginseng

Several types of plants are referred to as ginseng, but most studies of ginseng and diabetes have used American ginseng. Those studies have shown some glucose-lowering effects in fasting and post-prandial (after meal) blood glucose levels as well as in A1C levels (average blood glucose levels over a 3-month period). However, larger and more long-term studies are needed before general recommendations for use of ginseng can be made. Researchers also have determined that the amount of glucose-lowering compound in ginseng plants varies widely.

> **♣ It's A Fact!!**
> Although some people who use complementary or alternative therapies to treat diabetes may find the therapies effective, other therapies can be ineffective or even harmful.
>
> Source: National Diabetes Information Clearinghouse (NDIC).

Magnesium

Although the relationship between magnesium and diabetes has been studied for decades, it

✎ What's It Mean?

Insulin: A hormone that helps the body use glucose for energy. The beta cells of the pancreas make insulin. When the body cannot make enough insulin, insulin is taken by injection or through use of an insulin pump.

Pancreas: An organ that makes insulin and enzymes for digestion. The pancreas is located behind the lower part of the stomach and is about the size of a hand.

Type 1 Diabetes: A condition characterized by high blood glucose levels caused by a total lack of insulin. Occurs when the body's immune system attacks the insulin-producing beta cells in the pancreas and destroys them. The pancreas then produces little or no insulin. Type 1 diabetes develops most often in young people but can appear in adults.

Type 2 Diabetes: A condition characterized by high blood glucose levels caused by either a lack of insulin or the body's inability to use insulin efficiently. Type 2 diabetes develops most often in middle-aged and older adults but can appear in young people.

Source: "Diabetes Dictionary," National Diabetes Information Clearinghouse (NDIC), a service of the National Institute of Diabetes and Digestive and Kidney Diseases (NIDDK), National Institutes of Health (NIH), NIH Publication No. 06–3016, October 2005.

is not yet fully understood. Studies suggest that a deficiency in magnesium may worsen blood glucose control in type 2 diabetes. Scientists believe that a deficiency of magnesium interrupts insulin secretion in the pancreas and increases insulin resistance in the body's tissues. Evidence suggests that a deficiency of magnesium may contribute to certain diabetes complications. A recent analysis showed that people with higher dietary intakes of magnesium (through consumption of whole grains, nuts, and green leafy vegetables) had a decreased risk of type 2 diabetes.

Vanadium

Vanadium is a compound found in tiny amounts in plants and animals. Early studies showed that vanadium normalized blood glucose levels in animals with type 1 and type 2 diabetes. A recent study found that when people with diabetes were given vanadium, they developed a modest increase in insulin sensitivity and were able to decrease their insulin requirements. Currently researchers want to understand how vanadium works in the body, discover potential side effects, and establish safe dosages.

Chapter 55

Mental Health And Alternative Approaches

What Are Alternative Approaches To Mental Health Care?

An alternative approach to mental health care is one that emphasizes the interrelationship between mind, body, and spirit. Although some alternative approaches have a long history, many remain controversial. The National Center for Complementary and Alternative Medicine (NCCAM) at the National Institutes of Health was created in 1992 to help evaluate alternative methods of treatment and to integrate those that are effective into mainstream health care practice. It is crucial, however, to consult with your health care providers about the approaches you are using to achieve mental wellness.

Self-Help

Many people with mental illnesses find that self-help groups are an invaluable resource for recovery and for empowerment. Self-help generally refers to groups or meetings that:

• involve people who have similar needs;

About This Chapter: Information in this chapter is from "Alternative Approaches to Mental Health Care," National Mental Health Information Center, Substance Abuse and Mental Health Services Administration (SAMHSA), April 2003.

- are facilitated by a consumer, survivor, or other layperson;

- assist people to deal with a "life-disrupting" event, such as a death, abuse, serious accident, addiction, or diagnosis of a physical, emotional, or mental disability, for oneself or a relative;

- are operated on an informal, free-of-charge, and nonprofit basis;

- provide support and education; and

- are voluntary, anonymous, and confidential.

Diet And Nutrition

Adjusting both diet and nutrition may help some people with mental illnesses manage their symptoms and promote recovery. For example, research suggests that eliminating milk and wheat products can reduce the severity of symptoms for some people who have schizophrenia and some children with autism. Similarly, some holistic/natural physicians use herbal treatments, B-complex vitamins, riboflavin, magnesium, and thiamine to treat anxiety, autism, depression, drug-induced psychoses, and hyperactivity.

Pastoral Counseling

Some people prefer to seek help for mental health problems from their pastor, rabbi, or priest, rather than from therapists who are not affiliated with a religious community. Counselors working within traditional faith communities increasingly are recognizing the need to incorporate psychotherapy and/or medication, along with prayer and spirituality, to effectively help some people with mental disorders.

Animal Assisted Therapies

Working with an animal (or animals) under the guidance of a health care professional may benefit some people with mental illness by facilitating positive changes, such as increased empathy and enhanced socialization skills. Animals can be used as part of group therapy programs to encourage communication and increase the ability to focus. Developing self-esteem and reducing loneliness and anxiety are just some potential benefits of individual-animal therapy.

Expressive Therapies

Art Therapy: Drawing, painting, and sculpting help many people to reconcile inner conflicts, release deeply repressed emotions, and foster self-awareness, as well as personal growth. Some mental health providers use art therapy as both a diagnostic tool and as a way to help treat disorders such as depression, abuse-related trauma, and schizophrenia. You may be able to find a therapist in your area who has received special training and certification in art therapy.

Dance/Movement Therapy: Some people find that their spirits soar when they let their feet fly. Others, particularly those who prefer more structure or who feel they have "two left feet," gain the same sense of release and inner peace from the Eastern martial arts, such as aikido and tai chi. Those who are recovering from physical, sexual, or emotional abuse may find these techniques especially helpful for gaining a sense of ease with their own bodies. The underlying premise to dance/movement therapy is that it can help a person integrate the emotional, physical, and cognitive facets of "self."

Music/Sound Therapy: It is no coincidence that many people turn on soothing music to relax or snazzy tunes to help feel upbeat. Research suggests that music stimulates the body's natural "feel good" chemicals (opiates and endorphins). This stimulation results in improved blood flow, blood pressure, pulse rate, breathing, and posture changes. Music or sound therapy has been used to treat disorders such as stress, grief, depression, schizophrenia, and autism in children, and to diagnose mental health needs.

Culturally Based Healing Arts

Traditional Oriental medicine (such as acupuncture, shiatsu, and Reiki), Indian systems of health care (such as Ayurveda and yoga), and Native American healing practices (such as the sweat lodge and talking circles) all incorporate the following beliefs:

• Wellness is a state of balance between the spiritual, physical, and mental/emotional "selves."

• An imbalance of forces within the body is the cause of illness.

• Herbal/natural remedies, combined with sound nutrition, exercise, and meditation/prayer, will correct this imbalance.

Acupuncture: The Chinese practice of inserting needles into the body at specific points manipulates the body's flow of energy to balance the endocrine system. This manipulation regulates functions such as heart rate, body temperature, and respiration, as well as sleep patterns and emotional changes. Acupuncture has been used in clinics to assist people with substance abuse disorders through detoxification, to relieve stress and anxiety, to treat attention deficit and hyperactivity disorder in children, to reduce symptoms of depression, and to help people with physical ailments.

Ayurveda: Ayurvedic medicine is described as "knowledge of how to live." It incorporates an individualized regimen, such as diet, meditation, herbal preparations, or other techniques, to treat a variety of conditions, including depression, to facilitate lifestyle changes, and to teach people how to release stress and tension through yoga or transcendental meditation.

Yoga/meditation: Practitioners of this ancient Indian system of health care use breathing exercises, posture, stretches, and meditation to balance the body's energy centers. Yoga is used in combination with other treatment for depression, anxiety, and stress-related disorders.

Native American traditional practices: Ceremonial dances, chants, and cleansing rituals are part of Indian Health Service programs to heal depression, stress, trauma (including those related to physical and sexual abuse), and substance abuse.

Cuentos: Based on folktales, this form of therapy originated in Puerto Rico. The stories used contain healing themes and models of behavior such as self-transformation and endurance through adversity. Cuentos is used primarily to help Hispanic children recover from depression and other mental health problems related to leaving one's homeland and living in a foreign culture.

Relaxation And Stress Reduction Techniques

Biofeedback: Learning to control muscle tension and "involuntary" body functioning, such as heart rate and skin temperature, can be a path to mastering one's fears. It is used in combination with, or as an alternative to, medication to treat disorders such as anxiety, panic, and phobias. For example, a person can learn to "retrain" his or her breathing habits in stressful situations to induce relaxation and decrease hyperventilation. Some preliminary research indicates it may offer an additional tool for treating schizophrenia and depression.

Guided Imagery or visualization: This process involves going into a state of deep relaxation and creating a mental image of recovery and wellness. Physicians, nurses, and mental health providers occasionally use this approach to treat alcohol and drug addictions, depression, panic disorders, phobias, and stress.

Massage therapy: The underlying principle of this approach is that rubbing, kneading, brushing, and tapping a person's muscles can help release tension and pent-up emotions. It has been used to treat trauma-related depression and stress. A highly unregulated industry, certification for massage therapy varies widely from state to state. Some states have strict guidelines, while others have none.

Technology-Based Applications

The boom in electronic tools at home and in the office makes access to mental health information just a telephone call or a "mouse click" away. Technology is also making treatment more widely available in once-isolated areas.

Telemedicine: Plugging into video and computer technology is a relatively new innovation in health care. It allows both consumers and providers in remote or rural areas to gain access to mental health or specialty expertise. Telemedicine can enable consulting providers to speak to and observe patients directly. It also can be used in education and training programs for generalist clinicians.

Telephone counseling: Active listening skills are a hallmark of telephone counselors. These also provide information and referral to interested callers. For many people, telephone counseling often is a first step to receiving in-depth mental health care. Research shows that such counseling from specially trained mental health providers reaches many people who otherwise might not get the help they need. Before calling, be sure to check the telephone number for service fees; a 900 area code means you will be billed for the call, an 800 or 888 area code means the call is toll-free.

Electronic communications: Technologies such as the internet, bulletin boards, and electronic mail lists, provide access directly to consumers and the public on a wide range of information. On-line consumer groups can exchange information, experiences, and views on mental health, treatment systems, alternative medicine, and other related topics.

Radio psychiatry: Another relative newcomer to therapy, radio psychiatry was first introduced in the United States in 1976. Radio psychiatrists and psychologists provide advice, information, and referrals in response to a variety of mental health questions from callers. The American Psychiatric Association and the American Psychological Association have issued ethical guidelines for the role of psychiatrists and psychologists on radio shows.

✔ **Quick Tip**

This chapter does not cover every alternative approach to mental health. A range of other alternative approaches—psychodrama, hypnotherapy, recreational, and Outward Bound-type nature programs—offer opportunities to explore mental wellness. Before jumping into any alternative therapy, learn as much as you can about it. In addition to talking with your health care practitioner, you may want to visit your local library, bookstore, health food store, or holistic health care clinic for more information. Also, before receiving services, check to be sure the provider is properly certified by an appropriate accrediting agency.

Part Nine

If You Need More Information

Chapter 56

Getting Health Information From Trusted Sources

Government Agencies

There is a lot of information on complementary and alternative medicine (CAM), so it's important to go to sources you can trust. Good places to start are government agencies. They offer lots of information about CAM that might be helpful to you. They may also know of universities or hospitals that have CAM resources.

Be careful of products advertised by people or companies that:

* make claims that they have a "cure";

* do not give specific information about how well their product works;

* make claims only about positive results that have few side effects;

* say they have clinical studies, but provide no proof or copies of the studies.

Websites

Patients and families have been able to find answers to many of their questions about CAM on the internet. Many websites are good resources for CAM information. However, some may be unreliable or misleading.

About This Chapter: Information in this chapter is from "Getting Information from Trusted Sources," National Cancer Institute, U.S. National Institutes of Health, June 8, 2005.

These are questions to ask about a website:

- Who runs and pays for the site?

- Does it list any credentials?

- Does it represent an organization that is well known and respected?

- What is the purpose of the site, and who is it for?

- Is the site selling or promoting something?

- Where does the information come from?

- Is the information based on facts or only on someone's feelings or opinions?

- How is the information chosen? Is there a review board or do experts review the content?

- How current is the information?

- Does the site tell when it was last updated?

- How does the site choose which other sites to link you to?

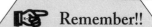
Remember!!
If a claim sounds too good to be true, it probably is.

Books

A number of books have been written about different CAM therapies. Some books are better than others and contain trustworthy content, while others do not.

If you go to the library, ask the staff for suggestions. Or if you live near a college or university, there may be a medical library available. Local bookstores may also have people on staff who can help you.

It's important to know that information is always changing and that new research results are reported every day. Be aware that if a book is written by only one person, you may only be getting that one person's view.

Here are some questions to ask:

- Is the author an expert on this subject?

- Do you know anyone else who has read the book?

- Has the book been reviewed by other experts?

- Was it published in the past 5 years?

- Does the book offer different points of view, or does it seem to hold one opinion?

- Has the author researched the topic in full?

- Are the references listed in the back?

Magazine Articles

If you want to look for articles you can trust, ask your librarian to help you look for medical journals, books, and other research that has been done by experts.

Articles in popular magazines are usually not written by experts. Rather, the authors speak with experts, gather information, and then write the article. If claims about CAM are made in magazine articles, remember the following:

- The authors may not have expert knowledge in this area.

- They may not say where they found their information.

- The articles have not been reviewed by experts.

- The publisher may have ties to advertisers or other organizations. Therefore, the article may be one-sided.

When you read these articles, you can use the same process that the magazine writer uses:

- Speak with experts.

- Ask lots of questions.

- Decide if the therapy is right for you.

Chapter 57

Fraudulent Health Claims: Don't Be Fooled

Whether they are looking for a short cut to losing weight or a cure for a serious ailment, consumers may be spending billions of dollars a year on unproven, fraudulently marketed, often useless health-related products, devices, and treatments. Why? Health fraud trades on false hope. It promises quick cures and easy solutions to a variety of problems, from obesity to cancer and AIDS; but consumers who fall for fraudulent "cure-all" products do not find help or better health. Instead, they find themselves cheated out of their money, their time, and maybe even their health. Fraudulently marketed health products can keep people from seeking and getting treatment from their own health care professional. Some products can cause serious harm, and many are expensive because health insurance rarely covers unapproved treatments.

To avoid becoming victims of health fraud, it's important for consumers to learn how to assess health claims and seek the advice of a health professional.

Common Health Fraud Targets

Officials at the Federal Trade Commission (FTC) and the Food and Drug Administration (FDA) say health fraud promoters often target people who are overweight or have serious conditions for which there are no cures,

About This Chapter: Information in this chapter is from "Miracle Health Claims: Add a Dose of Skepticism," U.S. Federal Trade Commission, September 2001.

including multiple sclerosis, diabetes, Alzheimer's disease, cancer, HIV and AIDS, and arthritis.

Cancer

A diagnosis of cancer can bring feelings of fear and hopelessness. Many people may be tempted to turn to unproven remedies promoted as cancer cures; but they and their loved ones should be skeptical of "miracle" claims because no single device, remedy, or treatment can treat all types of cancer. Cancer is a name given to a wide range of diseases; each requires different forms of treatment that are best determined with the advice of a health professional.

Cancer patients who want to try an experimental treatment should enroll in a legitimate clinical study. The FDA reviews clinical study designs to help ensure that patients are not subjected to unreasonable risks.

For more information about cancer treatments, contact the American Cancer Society; the nearest local chapter will be listed in the yellow pages of your phone book. For free publications on cancer research and treatment, call the National Cancer Institute's Cancer Information Service at 1-800-4-CANCER (1-800-422-6237) or log on to http://cancernet.nci .nih.gov/.

HIV And AIDS

Although legitimate treatments can extend life and improve the quality of life for people with AIDS, there is, so far, no cure for the disease. People diagnosed with HIV, the virus that causes AIDS, may want to try untested drugs or treatments; but trying unproven products or treatments, such as electrical and magnetic devices and so-called herbal cures, can be dangerous and may cause HIV-positive individuals to delay seeking medical care.

An example is the herb St. John's Wort, which has been promoted as a safe treatment for HIV. There is no evidence that this herb is effective in treating HIV, and in fact, studies have shown that it interferes with medicines prescribed for HIV.

People who think they may be HIV-positive may turn to home test kits; but claims for these products may be misleading and possibly harmful. Safe, reliable HIV testing can be done only through a medical professional or a clinic, or through the Home Access Express HIV-1 Test System; it is the only system approved for home use by the FDA.

The U.S. government has a toll-free HIV-AIDS Treatment Information Service, 1-800-HIV-0440 (1-800-448-0440), which is staffed by English- and Spanish-speaking health information specialists. Information also is available at www.hivatis.org.

Arthritis

Consumers spend an estimated $2 billion a year on unproven arthritis remedies—thousands of dietary and so-called natural cures, like mussel extract, desiccated liver pills, shark cartilage, CMO (cetylmyristoleate), honey and vinegar mixtures, and magnets and copper bracelets; but these remedies are not backed by adequate science to show that they offer long-term relief. For current, accurate information on arthritis treatments and alternative therapies, call the Arthritis Foundation at 1-800-283-7800 or visit its website at www.arthritis.org.

Assessing Claims For Dietary Supplements

The array of dietary supplements—vitamins and minerals, amino acids, enzymes, herbs, animal extracts and others—has grown tremendously over the years. Although the benefits of some of these products have been documented, the advantages of others are unproven.

For example, claims that a supplement allows you to eat all you want and lose weight effortlessly are false. To lose weight, you must lower your calorie intake or burn more calories—for example, by increasing exercise. Most medical experts recommend doing both.

Similarly, no supplement can cure arthritis or cancer in five days. Such claims are false. Consumers should be wary of any claims for a dietary supplement that say it can shrink tumors, cure insomnia, cure impotency, treat Alzheimer's disease, or prevent severe memory loss. These kinds of claims deal with the treatment of diseases, and companies that want to make such claims must follow the FDA's pre-market testing and review process required for new drugs.

Safety Concerns

Prescription drugs must undergo clinical testing and receive the FDA's full review for safety and effectiveness before they are sold. Over-the-counter medicines are subject to the OTC drug review process, which determines

♣ It's A Fact!!
FDA Regulation Of Health Claims

Federal law allows for certain claims to be made in the labeling of food and supplements. These include claims approved by the Food and Drug Administration that show a strong link, based on scientific evidence, between a food substance and a disease or health condition. These approved claims can state only that a food substance reduces the risk of certain health problems—not that it can treat or cure a disease. Two examples of approved claims are: "The vitamin folic acid may reduce the risk of neural tube defect-affected pregnancies," and "Calcium may reduce the risk of the bone disease osteoporosis."

Dietary supplements also may carry claims in their labeling that describe the effect of a substance in maintaining the body's normal structure or function, as long as the claims don't imply the product treats or cures a disease. The FDA does not review or authorize these claims. An example of such a claim is, "Product B promotes healthy joints and bones." When a dietary supplement is promoted with a claim like this, the claim must be accompanied with the disclaimer, "This statement has not been evaluated by the Food and Drug Administration. This product is not intended to diagnose, treat, cure, or prevent disease."

Source: Federal Trade Commission

safety and effectiveness of the products. Dietary supplements are not required to undergo government testing or review before they are marketed. Yet, supplements may have drug-like effects that could present risks for people on certain medicines or with certain medical conditions. This is true, even if the product is marketed as "natural." For example, St. John's Wort can have potentially dangerous interactions with a number of prescription drugs, including anticoagulants, oral contraceptives, antidepressants, antiseizure medicines, drugs for HIV, and drugs to prevent transplant rejection.

If you take a prescription medicine, always consult your health care professional before starting a dietary supplement.

Some dietary supplement substances require further scrutiny and study before they can be considered safe for all people. Though many supplements have a history of use, that history does not necessarily guarantee safety in every circumstance.

Some substances for which safety concerns have been raised are comfrey, chaparral, lobelia, germander, aristolochia, ephedra (ma huang), L-tryptophan, germanium, magnolia-stephania and stimulant laxative ingredients, such as those found in dieter's teas. The herb comfrey, for example, contains certain alkaloids that can cause serious liver damage. Consumers should not take any product containing comfrey either orally or as a suppository and should not apply comfrey products to broken skin.

Even some vitamins and minerals, when consumed in excessive quantities, can cause problems. For example, high intakes of vitamin A over a long period can reduce bone mineral density, cause birth defects, and lead to liver damage, according to the National Academy of Sciences.

To ensure the safe use of any health care product, read the labels and package inserts, follow product directions, and check with your health care professional.

How To Spot False Claims

When evaluating health-related claims, be skeptical. If something sounds too good to be true, it usually is. Here are some signs of a fraudulent claim:

- Statements that the product is a quick and effective cure-all or diagnostic tool for a wide variety of ailments. For example: "Extremely beneficial in the treatment of rheumatism, arthritis, infections, prostate problems, ulcers, cancer, heart trouble, hardening of the arteries, and more."

- Statements that suggest the product can treat or cure diseases. For example: "shrinks tumors" or "cures impotency."

- Promotions that use words like "scientific breakthrough," "miraculous cure," "exclusive product," "secret ingredient," or "ancient remedy." For example: "A revolutionary innovation formulated by using proven principles of natural health-based medical science."

- Text that uses impressive-sounding terms like these for a weight-loss product: "hunger stimulation point" and "thermo genesis."

- Undocumented case histories or personal testimonials by consumers or doctors claiming amazing results. For example: "My husband has Alzheimer's disease. He began eating a teaspoonful of this product each day, and now in just 22 days, he mowed the grass, cleaned out the garage, weeded the flower beds, and we take our morning walk again."

- Limited availability and advance payment requirements. For example: "Hurry. This offer will not last. Send us a check now to reserve your supply."

- Promises of no-risk "money-back guarantees." For example: "If after 30 days you have not lost at least 4 pounds each week, your uncashed check will be returned to you."

Avoiding Unscrupulous Dealers

It is easy to see why some people can be taken in by promoters' promises, especially when successful treatments have been elusive; but resist pressure to decide "on the spot" about trying an untested product or treatment. Ask for more information and consult a knowledgeable doctor, pharmacist, or other health care professional. Promoters of legitimate health care products do not object to your seeking additional information.

To learn whether the FDA or the FTC have taken action against the promoter of a product you may be considering, visit www.fda.gov/oc/enforcement.html or www.ftc.gov. Visit www.cfsan.fda.gov/~dms/ds -warn.html for a list of the dietary supplement ingredients for which the FDA has issued warnings.

In addition, if you're considering a clinic that requires you to travel and stay far from home for treatment, check it out with your doctor. Although some clinics offer effective treatments, others prescribe untested, unapproved, ineffective, and possibly dangerous "cures." In addition, the health care providers who work in these clinics may be unlicensed or lack other appropriate credentials.

For information about a particular hospital, clinic, or treatment center, contact the state or local health authorities where the facility is located. If the facility is in a foreign country, contact that government's health authority to see that the facility is properly licensed and equipped to handle the procedures involved. For information about facilities in Mexico, contact the Secretary of Health (Secretaria De Salud) in the Mexican state where the facility is located.

How To Report A Potential Problem

To report a health product that you believe is being advertised falsely, contact:

- the FTC by phone, toll-free, at 1-877-FTC-HELP (1-877-382-4357); TDD: 1-866-653-4261; by mail to Consumer Response Center, Federal Trade Commission, Washington, DC 20580; or online at www .ftc.gov. Click on "File a Complaint Online."

- your state Attorney General's office, state department of health, or local consumer protection agency. These offices are listed in the blue pages of your telephone book.

To report a product that you believe is fraudulently labeled, call your local FDA office. The number is listed in the blue pages of the telephone book.

♣ **It's A Fact!!**

Claims That Can Be Made For Conventional Foods And Dietary Supplements

Claims that can be used on food and dietary supplement labels fall into three categories: health claims, nutrient content claims, and structure/function claims. The responsibility for ensuring the validity of these claims rests with the manufacturer, FDA, or, in the case of advertising, with the Federal Trade Commission.

Health Claims

Health claims describe a relationship between a food, food component, or dietary supplement ingredient, and reducing risk of a disease or health-related condition. There are three ways by which FDA exercises its oversight in determining which health claims may be used on a label or in labeling for a food or dietary supplement: 1) the 1990 Nutrition Labeling and Education Act (NLEA) provides for FDA to issue regulations authorizing health claims for foods and dietary supplements after FDA's careful review of the scientific evidence submitted in health claim petitions; 2) the 1997 Food and Drug Administration Modernization Act (FDAMA) provides for health claims based on an authoritative statement of a scientific body of the U.S. government or the National Academy of Sciences; such claims may be used after submission of a health claim notification to FDA; and 3) the 2003 FDA Consumer Health Information for Better Nutrition Initiative provides for qualified health claims where the quality and strength of the scientific evidence falls below that required for FDA to issue an authorizing regulation. Such health claims must be qualified to assure accuracy and non-misleading presentation to consumers. The differences between these three methods of oversight for health claims are summarized below.

A "health claim" by definition has two essential components: 1) a substance (whether a food, food component, or dietary ingredient) and 2) a disease or health-related condition. A statement lacking either one of these components does not meet the regulatory definition of a health claim. For example, statements that address a role of dietary patterns or of general categories of foods (e.g., fruits and vegetables) in health are considered to be dietary guidance rather than health claims, provided that the context of the statement does not suggest that a specific substance is the subject. Dietary guidance statements used on food labels must be truthful and non-misleading. Statements that address a role of a specific substance in maintaining normal healthy structures or functions of the body are considered to be structure/function claims. Structure/function claims may not explicitly or implicitly link the relationship to a disease or health related condition. Unlike health claims, dietary guidance statements and structure/function claims are not subject to FDA review and authorization.

Nutrient Content Claims

The Nutrition Labeling and Education Act of 1990 (NLEA) permits the use of label claims that characterize the level of a nutrient in a food (i.e., nutrient content claims) made in accordance with FDA's authorizing regulations. Nutrient content claims describe the level of a nutrient or dietary substance in the product, using terms such as free, high, and low, or they compare the level of a nutrient in a food to that of another food, using terms such as more, reduced, and lite. An accurate quantitative statement (e.g., 200 mg of sodium) that does not "characterize" the nutrient level may be used to describe any amount of a nutrient present. However, a statement such as "only 200 mg of sodium" characterizes the level of sodium as being low and would therefore need to conform to the criteria of an appropriate nutrient content claim or carry a disclosure statement that it does not comply with the claim. Most nutrient content claim regulations apply only to those nutrients or dietary substances that have an established daily value: http://www.cfsan.fda.gov/~dms/flg-7a.html. The requirements that govern the use of nutrient content claims help ensure that descriptive terms, such as high or low, are used consistently for all types of food products and are thus meaningful to consumers. Healthy has been defined by a regulation as an implied nutrient content claim that characterizes a food that has "healthy" levels of total fat, saturated fat, cholesterol, and sodium. Percentage claims for dietary supplements are another category of nutrient content claims. These claims are used to describe a percentage level of a dietary ingredient for which there is no

Claims That Can Be Made For Conventional Foods And Dietary Supplements, continued

established Daily Value. Examples include simple percentage statements such as "40% omega-3 fatty acids, 10 mg per capsule," and comparative percentage claims, e.g., "twice the omega-3 fatty acids per capsule (80 mg) as in 100 mg of menhaden oil (40 mg)."

Structure/Function Claims

Structure/function claims have historically appeared on the labels of conventional foods and dietary supplements as well as drugs. However, the Dietary Supplement Health and Education Act of 1994 (DSHEA) established some special regulatory procedures for such claims for dietary supplement labels. Structure/function claims describe the role of a nutrient or dietary ingredient intended to affect normal structure or function in humans, for example, "calcium builds strong bones." In addition, they may characterize the means by which a nutrient or dietary ingredient acts to maintain such structure or function, for example, "fiber maintains bowel regularity," or "antioxidants maintain cell integrity," or they may describe general well-being from consumption of a nutrient or dietary ingredient. Structure/function claims may also describe a benefit related to a nutrient deficiency disease (like vitamin C and scurvy), as long as the statement also tells how widespread such a disease is in the United States. The manufacturer is responsible for ensuring the accuracy and truthfulness of these claims; they are not pre-approved by FDA but must be truthful and not misleading. If a dietary supplement label includes such a claim, it must state in a "disclaimer" that FDA has not evaluated the claim. The disclaimer must also state that the dietary supplement product is not intended to "diagnose, treat, cure, or prevent any disease," because only a drug can legally make such a claim. Manufacturers of dietary supplements that make structure/function claims on labels or in labeling must submit a notification to FDA no later than 30 days after marketing the dietary supplement that includes the text of the structure/function claim.

Source: U.S. Food and Drug Administration, CFSAN/Office of Nutritional Products, Labeling, and Dietary Supplements, September 2003.

To report an adverse reaction or illness that you think is related to the use of a supplement or other health care product, call a doctor or other health care provider immediately. You also may want to report your reaction or illness to FDA MedWatch. Call 1-800-FDA-1088 (1-800-332-1088) to request a report form, or file a complaint online at www.fda.gov/medwatch/report/hcp.htm. Patients' names are kept confidential. For more information on how to report a problem to FDA, see www.fda.gov/opacom/background ers/problem.html.

Food And Drug Administration

The FDA regulates over $1 trillion worth of products, which account for 25 cents of every dollar spent annually by American consumers. It is part of FDA's job to see that the food we eat is safe and wholesome and that the medicines and medical devices we use are safe and effective. For more information, call toll-free, 1-888-INFO-FDA (1-888-463-6332), or visit the FDA website, www.fda.gov.

Federal Trade Commission

The FTC works for the consumer to prevent fraudulent, deceptive, and unfair business practices in the marketplace and to provide information to help consumers spot, stop, and avoid them. To file a complaint or to get free information on consumer issues, visit www.ftc.gov or call toll-free, 1-877-FTC-HELP (1-877-382-4357); TTY: 1-866-653-4261. The FTC enters internet, telemarketing, identity theft, and other fraud-related complaints into Consumer Sentinel, a secure, online database available to hundreds of civil and criminal law enforcement agencies in the U.S. and abroad.

Chapter 58

How To Find Out If Your Insurance Covers CAM Treatments

How do patients pay for CAM treatments delivered by a practitioner?

In CAM, as in conventional medicine, there are two primary ways people pay for care:

- **Out-of-pocket payment.** Most consumers must pay for CAM practitioner services and CAM therapeutic products themselves.

- **Insurance.** Some health plans offer some coverage of CAM. Such coverage tends to be very limited, however, and varies considerably from state to state.

How can I find out if there are any laws in my state about insurance coverage of a CAM modality (treatment) that I am interested in?

There is no one central resource that collects this information for all the states. Some resources that may be helpful include the following:

- If you are seeking CAM treatment from a practitioner, there is likely to be one or more national professional associations for practitioners

About This Chapter: Information in this chapter is from "Consumer Financial Issues in Complementary and Alternative Medicine," National Center for Complementary and Alternative Medicine, NCCAM Publication No. D179, February 2005.

of that treatment—for example, associations for chiropractors. Many of these organizations monitor insurance coverage and reimbursement for their specialty. You can locate organizations by trying an internet search or asking a reference librarian for assistance.

- Each of the 50 states, as well as the District of Columbia and the four U.S. territories, has an agency that regulates the insurance industry in that state, enforces insurance laws, and assists consumers. This agency is often called the office of the state insurance commissioner. The services that this office provides vary by state, but each handles consumer inquiries. Your commissioner's office may be able to inform you of any requirements in your state for insurance coverage of a specific CAM modality.

I have health insurance. If I am interested in obtaining treatment from a CAM practitioner, what financial questions should I ask?

First, you need to be informed about your health insurance plan. Does it offer any coverage of CAM treatments? If so, what are the requirements and limits—for example, does the plan limit the conditions it will cover, require that CAM services be delivered by specific practitioners (such as a licensed medical doctor or a practitioner in the company's network), or cover only services that the plan determines to be medically necessary? Read your plan carefully, including the limits and exclusions. You may also want to check with the insurance company before you seek treatment.

Here are some questions to ask your insurer:

- Does this care need to be preauthorized or preapproved?

- Do I need a referral from my primary care provider? If so, be sure to obtain it and take it with you to the practitioner.

- What services, tests, or other costs will be covered?

- How many visits are covered and over what period of time?

- Is there a co-payment?

- Will the therapy be covered for any condition or only for certain conditions?

- Will any additional costs (for example, laboratory tests, dietary supplements, equipment, or supplies) be covered?

- Will I need to see a practitioner in your network? If so, can you provide me with a list of practitioners in my area?

- If I use a practitioner who is not part of your network, do you provide any coverage? Are there any additional out-of-pocket costs?

- Are there any dollar or calendar limits to my coverage?

What financial questions should I ask the practitioner?

Here are some questions to ask the practitioner or his office staff:

✔ **Quick Tip**

It will help you if you keep organized records about all interactions with your insurance company. Keep copies of letters, bills, and claims. Make notes about calls, including the date, time, customer service representative's name, and what you were told. If you are not satisfied with a representative's explanations, ask to speak to someone else.

- Do you accept my health insurance?

- Do I file the claim forms, or do you (the provider) take care of that?

- What is the cost for an initial appointment?

- How many treatments will I need?

- How much will each treatment cost?

- Can I receive treatment for a trial period to see if the therapy works for me before I commit to a full course?

- Will there be any additional costs?

It can also be useful to ask which insurance plans the practitioner accepts, in case you become interested in changing plans at some point (for example, through a change of employment).

What about CAM insurance coverage that may be offered through employers?

If CAM coverage is offered, it is usually one of the following types:

- **Higher deductibles.** A deductible is a total dollar amount that the consumer must pay before the insurer begins making payments for treatments. Under this type of policy, CAM coverage is offered, but the consumer pays a higher deductible.

- **Policy riders.** A rider is an amendment to an insurance policy that may change coverage in some way (such as increasing or decreasing benefits). You may be able to purchase a rider that adds or expands coverage in the area of CAM.

- **A contracted network of providers.** Some insurers work with a group of CAM providers who agree to offer services to group members at a rate lower than that offered to nonmembers. You pay out of pocket for treatment, but at a discounted rate.

> ✔ **Quick Tip**
>
> If you do not have insurance coverage for treatment, and paying the full fee each time would be difficult for you, you might ask:
>
> - Can your office arrange a payment plan so that my costs are spread out over a longer period of time?
>
> - Do you offer a sliding-scale fee? (A sliding-scale fee adjusts charges based on a patient's income and ability to pay.)

Employers negotiate with insurance companies for plan rates and services. This is done on a periodic basis (usually annually). You may wish to let your company's benefits administrator know about any coverage preferences you have. If your company offers more than one plan, evaluate carefully what each one offers, so you can pick the plan that best meets your needs.

The Agency for Healthcare Research and Quality (AHRQ), a federal agency, has helpful publications about choosing and using a health insurance plan.

Does NCCAM have a list of insurance companies that cover CAM?

As a medical research organization, NCCAM does not collect this kind of information and, therefore, does not have a list of companies that cover CAM. The following suggestions may be helpful:

- Talk to your family members, friends, and co-workers about their experiences with insurance companies and plans.

- Check what your state insurance commissioner's office has to offer. Many provide consumer publications, such as summaries of basic information about the health insurance companies operating in the state and/or ratings of those companies. Note that commissioners' offices do not provide recommendations or advice on specific companies.

- An insurance broker (an agent who sells policies for a variety of companies) may also be a resource.

My insurer has asked me for evidence, from scientific and medical literature, about the use of a CAM treatment. Can NCCAM provide this information?

The NCCAM Clearinghouse can help you find information from the scientific and medical literature on CAM. They use databases of peer-reviewed scientific and medical journals, such as CAM on PubMed. If you do not have access to the internet, the Clearinghouse can send information to you.

My insurance company has denied my claim for CAM treatment. Is there anything I can do?

Make sure you know your policy including what it is, and is not, supposed to cover. Health care providers and insurance companies use a standard set of codes in billing for medical services. Check whether there has been a coding error, either by the practitioner's office or by the insurance company; compare the codes on the practitioner's bill with the codes on the document you received from the insurance company. If you think your insurer made a mistake processing your claim, you can request a review from the company. Also, the insurance company should have an appeal procedure and provide a copy of it with your policy. It may be helpful to discuss with your practitioner whether he or she can do anything on your behalf, such as writing a letter. If you have taken these steps and the problem is not resolved, contact your state insurance commissioner's office, which has consumer complaint procedures.

Are there laws to help someone keep their health insurance during a job loss or job change? Do these laws apply to CAM treatments?

If you currently have an insurance plan that includes any CAM coverage, the following laws may be of interest to you.

The Health Insurance Portability and Accountability Act (HIPAA) of 1996 offers limited protections for many employed Americans. HIPAA protects health insurance coverage for workers and their families if the worker changes or loses his job. The law does the following:

- Limits the ability of insurance companies to refuse coverage based on preexisting conditions.

- Prevents group health plans from denying or charging more for coverage because of past or present poor health.

- Assures renewal of coverage, regardless of any health conditions of people covered under the policy.

- Guarantees certain small-business employers, and certain people who lose job-related coverage, the right to buy health insurance.

The Centers for Medicare and Medicaid Services can provide you with general information on the federal HIPAA program. Note that individual states may have specific laws related to HIPAA requirements; if you need more information on HIPAA in your state, contact your state insurance commissioner's office.

Another federal law that may help you is the Consolidated Omnibus Budget Reconciliation Act (COBRA) of 1985. COBRA continuation coverage gives you the chance to buy and maintain your current group health coverage for a defined period of time if you are laid off or have your work hours reduced below the level for receiving benefits. The length of continuation coverage depends on the reason for your loss of group coverage. COBRA generally covers health plans of businesses with 20 or more employees, employee organizations, and state or local governments. You must meet certain application deadlines and other conditions, such as payment schedules, to maintain coverage under COBRA. COBRA also can help you avoid a gap in coverage if you change jobs and are not immediately eligible for coverage in your new company.

For more information about COBRA, contact your nearest office of the Pension and Welfare Benefits Administration of the Department of Labor. Your state may also have a law that requires insurers to continue group plan coverage to individuals who lose their medical coverage for various reasons. Check with your state insurance commissioner's office.

What are tax-exempt accounts for medical expenses? How might they help me?

A flexible spending arrangement (FSA; sometimes called a Flexible Spending Account) is a benefit provided by some employers that offers a way to help pay for out-of-pocket medical expenses, while reducing the employee's taxable income. With FSAs for health-related expenses, you choose an amount of pre-tax dollars to be set aside from your paycheck each pay period. This money is then available to reimburse certain health-related expenses that are not paid any other way, such as by insurance. You may need to supply documentation from a physician or other health care provider that the treatment is medically necessary. Note that the IRS does not allow the same expense(s) to be both reimbursed through an FSA and claimed as a tax deduction.

Another type of tax-exempt benefit for health-related expenses is a health savings account (HSA). Set up by congress in December 2003, HSAs allow some individuals who participate in a high-deductible health plan to save money in a tax-free account. If you are eligible, you can use these savings to pay for your future medical expenses.

The IRS has publications with more information about FSAs and HSAs. The Department of the Treasury also has a direct link to information about HSAs on its website.

Does the federal government have resources that might help me financially with my health-related expenses?

Currently, federal health assistance programs are not set up to assist with CAM expenses specifically. They are intended to provide either direct support (direct payments) or indirect support (such as housing or child care credits, medical care at public clinics, or other social services) to people whom the government determines to be in need. Examples include people who meet the following criteria:

• Have a low income and limited resources

- Do not have other medical insurance

- Have a disability

- Are part of a population that has difficulty accessing medical care

- Are at least 65 years of age

- Have served in the military

There are federal databases on the internet that can introduce you to these programs. GovBenefits (www.govbenefits.gov) provides an overview and a self-test to help you identify whether any benefits are appropriate for your needs. FirstGov (www.firstgov.gov) has information on various health-related programs such as Medicare and Medicaid.

The Social Security Administration has two programs that pay benefits to people with disabilities:

- Social Security Disability Insurance (SSDI) pays benefits to disabled workers who have paid into Social Security through payroll deductions and to certain family members.

- Supplemental Security Income (SSI) pays benefits to people who are elderly or disabled and have low incomes.

The Department of Veterans Affairs may be able to help with health care costs if a family member served in the Armed Forces. Certain CAM treatments may be covered, such as chiropractic and acupuncture.

The Health Resources and Services Administration (HRSA) has several programs:

- While this program is not CAM-specific, the Hill-Burton program requires health care facilities (usually hospitals and clinics) that received certain federal funding to provide a specific amount of health care to needy persons free or at reduced cost. Eligibility is determined by income and family size, using the federal poverty guidelines.

- Through its Bureau of Primary Health Care (BPHC), HRSA funds community and migrant health care centers that treat people with limited access to medical services. Depending on the needs of the community, CAM care may be integrated with conventional care at these centers.

- Through the national "Insure Kids Now!" initiative, each state has a program to make health insurance available to infants, children, and teens in working families.

The Centers for Medicare and Medicaid Services, formerly the Health Care Financing Administration, administers the Medicare and Medicaid programs:

- **Medicare** is insurance for older persons and persons with disabilities. As of 2002, it includes some limited coverage of chiropractic services. Other CAM insurance coverage is under consideration.

- **Medicaid**, a joint federal-state program, is for people who need financial assistance for medical expenses. States may choose to provide optional Medicaid health care services, which could include CAM, in addition to required Medicaid services.

Also available through the Centers for Medicare and Medicaid Services is the State Children's Health Insurance Program, which expands health coverage to uninsured children in working families that earn too much for Medicaid but too little to afford private coverage.

The federal government also provides states and communities with various funds to assist needy persons, including medical care. To find out more about these benefits and whether you are eligible, contact your state or local department of social services. These departments are listed in the "Government" section of your phone book.

Some persons have inquired whether they can receive CAM treatments or financial assistance for treatments from NCCAM. Given its mission of research, training, and disseminating information, NCCAM does not provide financial assistance or treatment to consumers. As part of its research, NCCAM does conduct clinical trials of some CAM treatments (to find out more, go to http://nccam.nih.gov/clinicaltrials, or contact the NCCAM Clearinghouse).

Are CAM services deductible on income tax?

As of 2002, the IRS allows a limited number of deductibles for CAM services and products.

✔ **Quick Tip**

If treatment (whether CAM or conventional) for a disease or condition creates a financial crisis for you and your family, you may wish to try the following for more information:

• If you receive care at a hospital or clinic, that facility may have a social worker or patient advocate who can advise you.

• You may also find it helpful to contact nonprofit organizations that work on your disease or medical condition (try an internet search or check directories at your local library).

Chapter 59

Additional Reading About Complementary And Alternative Medicine

Books

Ayurveda: Nature's Medicine
Dr. David Frawley and Dr. Subhash Ranade
Lotus Press, Twin Lakes, WI, February 2001; ISBN: 0914955950

Becoming Vegetarian: The Essential Guide to a Healthy Vegetarian Diet
Vesanto Melina and Brenda Davis
Healthy Living Publications, Summertown, TN, August 2003; ISBN: 1570671443

The Best Alternative Medicine
Dr. Kenneth R. Pelletier
Fireside, New York, NY, March 2002; ISBN: 0743200276

About This Chapter: This chapter includes a compilation of various resources from many sources deemed reliable. It serves as a starting point for further research and is not intended to be comprehensive. Inclusion does not constitute endorsement. Resources in this chapter are categorized by type and, under each type, they are listed alphabetically by title to make topics easier to identify.

The Biblical Guide to Alternative Medicine
Dr. Neil T. Anderson and Dr. Michael Jacobson
Regal Books, Ventura, CA, January 2003; ISBN: 0830730834

The Chiropractic Way: How Chiropractic Care
Can Stop Your Pain and Help You Regain Your
Health Without Drugs or Surgery
Michael Lenarz
Bantam Dell, New York, NY, April 2003; ISBN: 0553381598

Complementary and Alternative Medicine Sourcebook:
Basic Consumer Health Information about Complementary
and Alternative Medical Therapies
Sandra J. Judd (Editor)
Omnigraphics, Inc., Detroit, MI, April 2006; ISBN: 0780808649

The Complete Body Massage Course: An Introduction
to the Most Popular Massage Therapies
Nicola Stewart
Collins & Brown, London, England, UK, March 2006; ISBN:
1843403196

The Guide to Complementary and Alternative
Medicine on the Internet
Lillian R. Brazin
The Haworth Press, Binghamton, NY, January 2004; ISBN: 0789015706

A Guide to Understanding Dietary Supplements
Shawn M. Talbott, PhD
The Haworth Press, Binghamton, NY, January 2003; ISBN: 0789014556

Healing Power of Acupressure and Acupuncture: A Complete
Guide to Timeless Traditions and Modern Practice
Matthew D. Bauer
Penguin Group, New York, NY, March 2005; ISBN: 1583332162

Healing Secrets of the Native Americans: Herbs, Remedies and Practices that Restore the Body, Refresh the Mind and Rebuild the Spirit

Porter Shimer

Black Dog & Leventhal Publishers, Inc., New York, NY, September 2004; ISBN: 1579123929

Herbs and Nutrients for the Mind: A Guide to Natural Brain Enhancers

Chris D. Meletis, N.D. and Jason E. Barker, N.D.

Praeger Publishers, Westport, CT, October 2004; ISBN: 0275983943

Homeopathy: Beyond Flat Earth Medicine

Timothy R. Dooley, N.D., M.D.

Timing Publications, San Diego, CA, October 2002; ISBN: 1886893012

Meditation As Medicine: Activate the Power of Your Natural Healing Force

Dharma Singh Khalsa, M.D.

Fireside, New York, NY, May 2002; ISBN: 0743400658

Nature Cures: The History of Alternative Medicine in America

James C. Whorton, PhD

Oxford University Press, USA, New York, NY, September 2002; ISBN: 0195140710

The Reflexology Atlas

Bernard C. Kolster, M.D. and Astrid Waskowiak, M.D.

Healing Arts Press, Rochester, VT, December 2005; ISBN: 1594770913

The Rolfing Experience: Integration in the Gravity Field

Betsy Sise

Hohm Press, Prescott, AZ, November 2005; ISBN: 1890772526

Articles

"Ayurvedic Medicine: Meaning 'science of life' in Sanskrit, this 5,000-year-old healing system is right in sync with our growing awareness of the mind-body connection," by Jill Neimark, *Natural Health*, June 2004, p. 76(6).

"Complementary and Alternative Medicine," *World Almanac and Book of Facts*, Annual 2004, p. 530.

"Complementary and Alternative Medicine: Is there a fit in behavioral health?" by Jeanne Supin, *Behavioral Healthcare Tomorrow*, December 2005, p. 17(5).

"Got Flex? There's a new way to exercise, and it's muscling its way into a gym near you," by Monica Smith, *Current Health 2*, November 2005, p. 24(3).

"Hands-On Health with Reflexology," by Kate Worfolk, *Natural Life*, January-February 2006, p. 10(3).

"Healthy Living: Americans turning to complementary and alternative medicine," *Fort Worth Star-Telegram*, August 23, 2004, p. NA.

"The Homeopathy Guide: This classic mind/body therapy uses tiny doses of natural substances to help your body's own healing energies overcome illness and restore balance," by Tom Weede, *Natural Health*, April 2005, p. 74(6).

"Hospitals Get Alternative," *U.S. News & World Report*, July 22, 2002, p. 68.

"How to Lift the Mind: For those suffering from the pain of anxiety and depression, complementary medicine is no miracle cure. But some treatments offer real hope," by Claudia Kalb, *Newsweek*, December 2, 2002, p. 67.

"Hypnosis: A safe and potent pain reliever," *Consumer Reports*, January 2005, p. 49(1).

"Light Therapy for Winter Depression," *Harvard Women's Health Watch*, February 2005, p. NA.

"Naturopathic Medicine," by Beth Wotton, *American Fitness*, January-February 2004, p. 8(2).

"Now, Integrative Care," by Geoffrey Cowley, *Newsweek*, December 2, 2002, p. 46.

"Nutrition from the Kitchen, Not the Lab: Tufts researchers conclude that eating right is still smarter than relying on supplements," *Tufts University Health & Nutrition Letter*, November 2005, p. 1(2).

"The Power Within: Tap into your own energy reserves with top strategies from Ayurveda, Reiki, hypnotherapy, and TCM," by Suz Redfearn, *Natural Health*, February 2005, p. 67(5).

"Three Popular Nutritional Supplements Do Not Work," *HealthFacts*, March 2006, p. 5.

"Use of Complementary and Alternative Medicine," *Nutrition Research Newsletter*, May 2002, p. 14(2).

"What Chiropractors Can and Can't Do For You," *Tufts University Health & Nutrition Letter*, February 2003, p. 8(1).

Web Page Documents

Botanical Supplements: Weeding Out the Health Risks
National Institute of Environmental Health Sciences
http://ehp.niehs.nih.gov/members/2004/112-13/spheres.html

Chiropractic
WholeHealth Chicago
http://www.wholehealthchicago.com/chiropractic.htm

Complementary and Alternative Medicine: What is it?
Mayo Foundation for Medical Education and Research
http://www.mayoclinic.com/health/alternative-medicine/PN00001

Frequently Asked Questions About Acupuncture
American Academy of Medical Acupuncture
http://www.medicalacuppuncture.org/acu_info/faqs.html

Herbal Products and Supplements: What You Should Know
American Academy of Family Physicians
http://familydoctor.org/860.xml?printxml

Meditation Study Shows Life Gains
U.S. Department of Health and Human Services
http://www.healthfinder.gov/news/newsstory.asp?docid=525444

More Than One-Third of U.S. Adults Use Complementary and Alternative Medicine, According to New Government Survey
Centers for Disease Control and Prevention
http://www.cdc.gov/nchs/pressroom/04news/adultsmedicine.htm

Music Therapy
Association of Professional Music Therapists
http://www.apmt.org/mt-whatismt.htm

A Natural Product Does Not Mean a Safe Product
National Cancer Institute
http://www.cancer.gov/cancertopics/thinking-about-CAM/page7

Reiki, Questions and Answers
The International Center for Reiki Training
http://www.reiki.org/FAQ/Questions&Answers.html

Seasonal Affective Disorder and Light Therapy
The Cleveland Clinic
http://www.clevelandclinic.org/health/health-info/docs/1400/
1484.asp?index=6412

T'ai Chi
The Nemours Foundation
http://kidshealth.org/teen/food_fitness/exercise/tai_chi.html

Therapeutic Touch
Hartford Hospital
http://www.harthosp.org/IntMed/tt.htm

Using Complementary Therapy to Relieve Pain
The National Pain Foundation
http://www.nationalpainfoundation.org/MyTreatment/
News_Complementary.asp

What is a Doctor of Osteopathic Medicine (D.O.)
American Osteopathic Association
http://www.osteopathic.org/index.cfm?PageID=ado_whatis

What is homeopathy?
National Center for Homeopathy
http://www.homeopathic.org/whatis.htm

Yoga
The Nemours Foundation
http://kidshealth.org/teen/food_fitness/exercise/yoga.html

Chapter 60

Complementary And Alternative Medicine: A Directory Of Resources

National Organizations

Alternative Medicine Foundation, Inc.

P.O. Box 60016
Potomac, MD 20859
Phone: 301-340-1960
Fax: 301-340-1936
Website: http://
www.amfoundation.org
E-mail: info@amfoundation.org

American Academy of Medical Acupuncture (AAMA)

4929 Wilshire Boulevard, Suite 428
Los Angeles, CA 90010
Phone: 323-937-5514
Website: http://
www.medicalacupuncture.org
E-mail: JDOWDEN@prodigy.net

American Art Therapy Association, Inc.

5999 Stevenson Ave.
Alexandria, VA 22304
Toll Free: 888-290-0878
Website:
http://www.arttherapy.org
E-mail: info@arttherapy.org

About This Chapter: Information in this chapter was compiled from many sources deemed reliable; inclusion does not constitute endorsement. All contact information was verified and updated in March 2006.

American Association of Colleges of Osteopathic Medicine

5550 Friendship Blvd., Suite 310
Chevy Chase, MD 20815-7231
Phone: 301-968-4100
Fax: 301-968-4101
Website: http://www.aacom.org

American Association of Naturopathic Physicians

4435 Wisconsin Ave., NW, Suite 403
Washington, DC 20016
Toll Free: 866-538-2267
Phone: 202-237-8150
Fax: 202-237-8152
Website: http://www.naturopathic.org
E-mail:
member.services@Naturopathic.org

American Association of Oriental Medicine

P.O. Box 162340
Sacramento, CA 95816
Toll Free: 866-455-7999
Phone: 916-443-4770
Fax: 916-443-4766
Website: http://www.aaom.org

American Association of Professional Hypnotherapists

4149-A El Camino way
Palo Alto, CA 94306
Phone: 650-323-3224
Website: http://www.aaph.org

American Chiropractic Association

1701 Clarendon Boulevard
Arlington, VA 22209
Toll Free: 800-896-4643
Phone: 703-276-8800
Fax: 703-243-2593
Website: http://www.amerchiro.org
E-mail: memberinfo@acatoday.org

American Dance Therapy Association, Inc.

2000 Century Plaza, Suite 108
10632 Little Patuxent Parkway
Columbia, MD 21044
Phone: 410-997-4040
Fax: 410-997-4048
Website: http://www.adta.org
E-mail: info@adta.org

American Holistic Medical Association

12101 Menaul Blvd., NE, Suite C
Albuquerque, NM 87112
Phone: 505-292-7788
Fax: 505-293-7582
Website: http://
www.holisticmedicine.org
E-mail:
ksummers@holisticmedicine.org

American Massage Therapy Association

500 Davis Street, Suite 900
Evanston, IL 60201-4695
Toll Free: 877-905-2700
Phone: 847-864-0123
Fax: 847-864-1178
Website: http://
www.amtamassage.org
E-mail: info@amtamassage.org

American Meditation Institute

60 Garner Road, P.O. Box 430
Averill Park, NY 12018
Toll Free: 800-234-5115
Phone: 518-674-8714
Fax: 518-674-8714
Website: http://
www.americanmeditation.org
E-mail:
ami@americanmeditation.org

American Music Therapy Association, Inc.

8455 Colesville Road, Suite 1000
Silver Spring, MD 20910
Phone: 301-589-3300
Fax: 301-589-5175
Website: http://
www.musictherapy.org
E-mail: info@musictherapy.org

American Osteopathic Association

142 East Ontario Street
Chicago, IL 60611
Toll Free: 800-621-1773
Phone: 312-202-8000
Fax: 312-202-8200
Website: http://www.osteopathic.org

American Reflexology Certification Board

P.O. Box 740879
Arvada, CO 80006-0879
Phone: 303-933-6921
Fax: 303-904-0460
Website: http://www.arcb.net
E-mail: info@arcb.net

American Society of Clinical Hypnosis

140 N. Bloomingdale Rd.
Bloomingdale, IL 60108-1017
Phone: 630-980-4740
Fax: 630-351-8490
Website: http://www.asch.net
E-mail: info@asch.net

Association for Applied Psychophysiology and Biofeedback

10200 West 44th Avenue, Suite 304
Wheat Ridge, CO 80033
Toll Free: 800-477-8892
Phone: 303-422-8436
Website: http://www.aapb.org
E-mail: aapb@resourcenter.com

Center for Mind-Body Medicine

5225 Connecticut Ave., NW
Suite 414
Washington, DC 20015
Phone: 202-966-7338
Fax: 202-966-2589
Website: http://www.cmbm.org
E-mail: center@cmbm.org

International Center for Reiki Training

21421 Hilltop Street, Unit #28
Southfield, MI 48034
Toll Free: 800-332-8112
Phone: 248-948-8112
Fax: 248-948-9534
Website: http://www.reiki.org
E-mail: center@reiki.org

International Chiropractors Association

1110 N. Glebe Rd., Suite 650
Arlington, VA 22201
Toll Free: 800-423-4690
Phone: 703-528-5000
Fax: 703-528-5023
Website: http://
www.chiropractic.org

National Association for Holistic Aromatherapy

3327 W. Indian Trail Road
PMB 144
Spokane, WA 99208
Toll Free: 888-275-6242
Phone: 509-325-3419
Fax: 509-325-3479
Website: http://www.naha.org
E-mail: info@naha.org

National Ayurvedic Medical Association

620 Cabrillo Avenue
Santa Cruz, CA 95065
Website:
http://www.ayurveda-nama.org
E-mail: info@ayurveda-nama.org

National Center for Complementary and Alternative Medicine

NCCAM Clearinghouse
P.O. Box 7923
Gaithersburg, MD 20898
Toll Free: 888-644-6226
Phone: 301-519-3153
TTY: 866-464-3615
Fax: 866-464-3616
Website: http://nccam.nih.gov
E-mail: info@nccam.nih.gov

National Certification Commission for Acupuncture and Oriental Medicine

11 Canal Center Plaza, Suite 300
Alexandria, VA 22314
Phone: 703-548-9004
Fax: 703-548-9079
Website: http://www.nccaom.org
E-mail: info@nccaom.org

National Institute of Ayurvedic Medicine

375 5th Avenue, 5th Floor
New York, NY 10016
Phone: 845-278-8700
or 212-685-8600
Fax: 845-278-8215
Website: http://www.niam.com
E-mail: ayurveda@niam.com

National Qigong Association

P.O. Box 252
Lakeland, MN 55043
Toll Free: 888-815-1893
Website: http://www.nqa.org
E-mail: info@nqa.org

Office of Cancer Complementary and Alternative Medicine (OCCAM)

National Cancer Institute
6116 Executive Blvd., Suite 609,
MSC 8339
Bethesda, MD 20892
Toll Free: 800-4CANCER
Clearinghouse: 888-644-6226
Website: http://www.cancer.gov/cam

Office of Dietary Supplements

National Institutes of Health
6100 Executive Blvd., Room 3B01,
MSC 7517
Bethesda, MD 20892-7517
Phone: 301-435-2920
Fax: 301-480-1845
Website: http://
www.ods.od.nih.gov
E-mail: ods@nih.gov

Qigong Institute

561 Berkeley Avenue
Menlo Park, CA 94025
Website: http://
www.qigonginstitute.org

Reflexology Association of
America
P.O. Box 26744
Columbus, OH 43226-0744
Phone: 740-657-1695
Fax: 740-657-1695
Website:
http://www.reflexology-usa.org

Rolf Institute of Structural
Integration
5055 Chaparral Ct., Suite 103
Boulder, CO 80301
Toll Free: 800-530-8875
Phone: 303-449-5903
Fax: 303-449-5978
Website: http://www.rolf.org
E-mail: info@rolf.org

Society for Light Treatment
and Biological Rhythms
4648 Main Street
Chincoteague, VA 23336
Fax: 757-336-5777
Website: http://www.sltbr.org
E-mail: sltbrinfo@aol.com

U.S. Food and Drug
Administration
5600 Fishers Lane
Rockville, MD 20857
Toll Free: 888-INFO-FDA (888-463-6332)
Website: http://www.fda.gov

Internet Resources

Chinese Medicine Sampler
http://www.chinesemedicinesampler.com

Food and Nutrition Information Center—Alternative Medicine
http://www.nal.usda.gov/fnic/etext/ds_altmed.html

HerbMed
http://www.herbmed.org

Home of Reflexology
http://www.reflexology.org

Information Resource: About Herbs, Botanicals and Other Products—Memorial Sloan Kettering Cancer Center
http://www.mskcc.org/aboutherbs

International Bibliographic Information on Dietary Supplements (IBIDS) Database
http://dietary-supplements.info.nih.gov/Health_Information/IBIDS.aspx

Jiva Ayurveda
http://www.ayurvedic.org

MayoClinic.com—Complementary and Alternative Medicine
http://www.mayoclinic.com/health/alternative-medicine/CM99999

Medicinal Herb Garden—University of Washington
http://nnlm.gov/pnr/uwmhg

MedlinePlus—Complementary and Alternative Therapies Topics
http://www.nlm.nih.gov/medlineplus/
complementaryandalternativetherapies.html

NOAH-Complementary and Alternative Medicine
http://www.noah-health.org/en/alternative

Quackwatch
http://www.quackwatch.org

Index

Page numbers that appear in *Italics* refer to illustrations. Page numbers that have a small 'n' after the page number refer to information shown as Notes at the beginning of each chapter. Page numbers that appear in **Bold** refer to information contained in boxes on that page (except Notes information at the beginning of each chapter).

A

AAFP *see* American Academy of Family Physicians
AAMA *see* American Academy of Medical Acupuncture
"About Art Therapy" (American Art Therapy Association, Inc.) 289n
"About Chiropractic and Its Use in Treating Low-Back Pain" (NCCAM) 111n
"About Reflexology" (Association of Reflexologists) 135n
accreditation *see* certification
acquired immune deficiency syndrome (AIDS), fraudulent claims 354–55
acupressure
overview 91–94
safety concerns **93**
"Acupressure" (WholeHealth Chicago) 91n
acupuncture
versus acupressure 92
cancer treatment 332–33
defined **73, 116**
described 32–33

acupuncture, continued
diabetes mellitus 337
mental health 344
overview 95–100
pain management 319
traditional Chinese medicine 74, 76
"Acupuncture" (NCCAM) 95n
"Acupuncture As A Cancer Treatment" (NCI) 329n
"Acupuncture PDQ: Complementary and Alternative Medicine - Patient" (NCI) 329n
A.D.A.M., Inc., publications
biofeedback 191n
mind-body medicine 185n
tai chi 223n
therapeutic touch 277n
yoga 227n
adjustments, chiropractic 114
see also chiropractic medicine
AIDS *see* acquired immune deficiency syndrome
alcohol abuse, biofeedback 193
Alexander, Frederick Matthias 101

Alexander technique
  defined 86
  goal 102
  overview 101–3
"Alexander Technique"
  (WholeHealth Chicago) 101n
allopathic physicians, applied
  kinesiology 109
alternating current field therapy,
  described 5
"Alternative Approaches to Mental
  Health Care" (SAMHSA) 341n
alternative medicine
  described 3–4
  doctor opinions 18–19
Alternative Medicine Foundation, Inc.,
  contact information 383
American Academy of Family Physicians
  (AAFP), Web site address 380
American Academy of Medical
  Acupuncture (AAMA)
  contact information 383
  Web site address 379
American Apitherapy Society, Inc.,
  apitherapy publication 235n
American Art Therapy Association, Inc.
  art therapy publication 289n
  contact information 383
American Association for Applied and
  Therapeutic Humor, contact
  information 300
American Association of Colleges of
  Osteopathic Medicine
  contact information 384
  osteopathic medicine publication 67n
American Association of Naturopathic
  Physicians
  contact information 384
  naturopathic medicine publication 59n
American Association of Oriental
  Medicine, contact information 384
American Association of Professional
  Hypnotherapists, contact
  information 384
American Chiropractic Association,
  contact information 384
American Dance Therapy Association
  contact information 384
  dance/movement therapy publication 293n

American Heart Association, chelation
  therapy publication 239n
American Holistic Medical Association,
  contact information 384
American Indian medicine see traditional
  Native American medicine
American Massage Therapy Association,
  contact information 385
American Meditation Institute, contact
  information 385
American Music Therapy Association
  contact information 385
  music therapy publication 311n
American Osteopathic Association
  contact information 385
  Web site address 381
American Reflexology Certification
  Board, contact information 385
American Society of Clinical Hypnosis
  contact information 385
  hypnosis information publication 201n
amethyst, described 246
amino acids, defined 154
Angelou, Virginia 195n
animal assisted therapies, mental
  health 342
anmo 76
anxiety, CAM therapies 11
apitherapy
  experimentation 237
  overview 235–37
applied kinesiology
  history 106
  overview 105–10
"Applied Kinesiology Logo"
  (ICAK-USA) 105n
aquamarine, described 246
"Are Detox Diets Safe?" (Nemours
  Foundation) 165n
"Are You Considering Using
  Complementary and Alternative
  Medicine (CAM)?" (NCCAM) 13n
arogyawardhini 46
aromatherapy
  described 288
  guided imagery 198
  overview 285–88
"Aromatherapy" (Better Health
  Channel) 285n

Artemisia annua 33–34
arthritis
  CAM therapies *11*
  fraudulent claims 355
art therapy
  mental health 343
  overview 289–90
  reputation **290**
asanas, described 230
Association for Applied
  Psychophysiology and Biofeedback,
  contact information 385
Association of Cancer Online Resources,
  cancer pain publication 317n
Association of Professional Music
  Therapists, Web site address 380
Association of Reflexologists, reflexology
  publication 135n
Astanga yoga, described 228
Aston, Judith 141
atherosclerosis, chelation therapy 239–40
atopic dermatitis, traditional Chinese
  medicine 76
attunements, Reiki 271–72, 275
autogenic training, described 186–87
autonomous nervous system,
  described 212
ayur, defined 39
ayurvedic medicine
  active participation **42**
  cautions **49**
  described 34
  mental health 344
  overview 39–50
  treatment goals **44**

B

back pain, CAM therapies *11*
bacteria *see* probiotics
balance
  acupuncture 98
  ayurvedic medicine **40, 42, 49**
  doshas 43
  homeopathy **52**
  mental health 343–44
  reflexology 135, 136
  traditional Chinese medicine 31–32,
    33, 72

balance, continued
  traditional Native American
    medicine 79–80, **80**
  yoga 227, 229
Barnes, Vernon A. **210**
bee venom *see* apitherapy
beliefs, treatment effectiveness 15
Benson, Herbert 186
Better Health Channel, aromatherapy
  publication 285n
Bhakti yoga, described 228
Bikram yoga, described 228
bioelectromagnetic-based therapies,
  described 5
biofeedback
  described 186, 189
  diabetes mellitus 338
  disorders treatment **192**
  mental health 344–45
  overview 191–94
  pain management 319
"Biofeedback" (A.D.A.M., Inc.) 191n
biologically based therapies, described 4
black cohosh 152
Blackman, Janine **18–19**
bladder control, biofeedback 193
bloodletting, defined **58**
bloodstone, described 246
Bode, Anne 243n
body-based therapies
  described 5
  overview 85–90
Bonakdar, Roberts **18–19**
boswellia 50
"Botanical Dietary Supplements:
  Background Information"
  (NIH) 157n
botanical medicine, described 64
botanicals, defined **154**
botanical supplements
  overview 156–63
  safety concerns **160–61**
  see also dietary supplements
Breitbart, William 218

C

cadmium 58
calcite, described 246

calcium
  chelation therapy 240
  vegetarianism 180
California Research Foundation,
  probiotics publication 255n
CAM *see* complementary and
  alternative medicine
CAM therapies
  cancer 329–36
  diabetes mellitus 337–40
  overview 3–5
  statistics 7–12
cancer
  CAM therapies 329–36
  fraudulent claims 354
"Cancer Pain Treatments: Alternative/
  Complementary Methods" (Association
  of Cancer Online Resources) 317n
Caraka Samhita 40
carnelian, described 246
cauda equina syndrome, defined **116**
CDC *see* Centers for Disease
  Control and Prevention
celiac disease, defined **252**
cellulase 249
Center for Mind-Body Medicine,
  contact information 386
Centers for Disease Control and
  Prevention (CDC), Web site
  address 380
central nervous system (CNS)
  acupuncture 33
  craniosacral therapy 121
certification
  acupuncture practitioners 78, **98**, 99
  Alexander technique 103
  applied kinesiology 107–8
  art therapists 290
  ayurvedic practitioners 46
  CAM practitioners 20–21, 24
  chiropractors 112–14
  dance therapists 294
  enzyme therapy 253
  health spas **127**
  homeopathic practitioners 54–55
  humor therapists 300
  hypnotherapists 203–4
  massage therapists 133–34
  osteopathic physicians 67–68

certification, continued
  reflexology 137
  Reiki teachers **274**
  therapeutic touch 281
Chace, Marian 293
chakras, crystal therapy 244–45
cheir, defined 111
chelation therapy, overview 239–42
chi kung *see* qigong
childbirth, naturopathic medicine 65
Chinese herbs, described **74**
Chinese Materia Medica, described 32,
  33–34
Chinese medicine *see* traditional
  Chinese medicine
Chinese Medicine Sampler, Web site
  address 388
Chinese Thunder God vine 34
chiropractic medicine
  defined **73**, 86
  non-manual treatments **115**
  overview 111–19
  statistics *11*, 85
  training, described **113**
chromium 152, 338
cinchona bark 52
citrine, described 246
clear quartz, described 246
Cleveland Clinic, Web site address 380
clinical trials
  acupuncture 32–33
  ayurvedic medicine 34, 48
  cancer treatment 331, **331**
  chiropractic 115–18
  defined **116**
  homeopathic remedies 57
  homeopathy 36
  manipulative therapies 87, 88
  Thunder God vine 34
cognitive behavioral therapy
  described 186
  pain management 318
cold compresses 128
cold therapy 127
  see also hydrotherapy
colonic irrigation
  defined **166**
  safety concerns **126**
  see also enema

Commiphora mukul 46
"Complementary and Alternative Medical
  Therapies for Diabetes" (NIDDK) 337n
complementary and alternative medicine
  (CAM)
  overview 3–5
  statistics 7–12
complementary medicine, described 3
compresses 128
constitution, ayurvedic medicine 41–42
"Consumer Financial Issues in
  Complementary and Alternative
  Medicine" (NCCAM) 365n
controlled clinical trial, defined **116**
Cooke, David A. 301n, 317n
cowhage 50
craniosacral therapy
  defined **86**
  overview 121–24
credentials *see* certification
Creighton University School of Medicine,
  magnet therapy publication 263n
crystal therapy
  energy **244**
  healing energy **248**
  overview 243–48
"Crystal Therapy" (Bode) 243n
cuentos, mental health 344
curcuminoids 50
cystic fibrosis, defined **252**

D

DanActive 260
"Dance/Movement Therapy" (American
  Dance Therapy Association) 293n
dance therapy
  disease prevention **294**
  mental health 343
  overview 293–95
dandelion, described **159**
decoction, described 158
deep breathing, statistics *11*
Department of Health and Human
  Services (DHHS; HHS) *see* US
  Department of Health and Human
  Services
Department of Labor (DOL) *see* US
  Department of Labor

depression
  applied kinesiology 110
  CAM therapies *11*
  magnetic therapy 266–67
detox diet, overview 165–68
DHHS *see* US Department of Health
  and Human Services
diabetes mellitus, CAM therapies
  337–40, **338**
diamond, described 246
diet and nutrition
  applied kinesiology 105, 109
  ayurvedic medicine 44, 45–46
  mental health 342
  naturopathic medicine 64
  probiotics 255–62
  see also detox diet; macrobiotic diet;
    raw food diet; vegetarian diets
Dietary Supplement Health and
  Education Act (1994) 157
dietary supplements
  applied kinesiology 108
  ayurvedic medicine 48
  described **47**
  enzyme therapy 249
  fraudulent claims 355–56
  overview 145–55
  probiotics **259**
  regulation 15, **356, 360–62**
  see also botanical supplements
diets, statistics *11*
direct current field therapy, described 5
disease resistance, craniosacral therapy **122**
distraction, pain management 318
DO *see* osteopathic medicine
DOL *see* US Department of Labor
doshas 42–44
drug interactions, dietary
  supplements **148**
duodenum, defined **252**

E

echinacea 35, 152
echocardiography, blood pressure **210**
ECT *see* electroconvulsive therapy
eczema, traditional Chinese medicine 77
EDAD *see* endothelial-dependent arterial
  dilation

EDTA (ethylenediamine
tetraacetic acid) 240–42
EEG *see* electroencephalography
electroconvulsive therapy (ECT),
defined 266
electroencephalography (EEG),
described 192
electromagnetic field therapy, described 5
electromyography (EMG), described 191
emerald, described 247
EMG *see* electromyography
endorphins, acupuncture 33
endothelial-dependent arterial dilation
(EDAD), meditation 211
endothelium, described 210
enema, defined 166
energy, crystals 244
see also qi
energy therapies, described 5
enzymes, defined 154
"Enzyme Therapy" (Gale Group)
249n
enzyme therapy, overview 249–53
ephedra, FDA ban 150–51
ephedrine 150–51
epilepsy, aromatherapy 288
essential oils
aromatherapy 286–87
cautions 288
defined 236
"An Exploration of Guided Imagery
and Visualization" (Angelou) 195n
extract, described 158

F

Fabry's disease, enzyme therapy 251
fasting, detox diets 167–68
FDA *see* US Food and Drug
Administration
Federal Trade Commission (FTC)
see US Federal Trade Commission
fibromyalgia, defined 97
financial considerations
CAM therapies 12, 24, 25
chelation therapy 240–41
crisis information 374
light therapy 307–8
magnet therapy 267

financial considerations, continued
manipulative therapies 89–90
payment plans 368
Reiki 275
Fitzgerald, William 136
Flexner Report 53
folic acid 146
Food, Drug and Cosmetic Act 150
Food and Drug Administration
(FDA) *see* US Food and Drug
Administration
Food and Nutrition Information
Center, Web site address 388
foot massage *see* massage therapy;
reflexology
forms, tai chi 225
fraud
complementary and alternative
medicine 16–17
overview 353–63
"Frequently Asked Question and
Consumer Information" (California
Research Foundation) 255n
"Frequently Asked Questions"
(Association of Reflexologists) 135n
"Frequently Asked Questions About
Apitherapy" (American Apitherapy
Society, Inc.) 235n
"Frequently Asked Questions About Art
Therapy" (American Art Therapy
Association, Inc.) 289n
"Frequently Asked Questions about
CranioSacral Therapy" (Upledger
Institute, Inc.) 121n
"Frequently Asked Questions
About Music Therapy" (American
Music Therapy Association) 311n
friction rubs 128
FTC *see* US Federal Trade Commission

G

Gale Group, enzyme therapy
publication 249n
garlic 153
garnet, described 247
Gaucher's disease, defined 252
gemstone therapy, overview 243–48
general review, defined 116

"Getting Information from Trusted Sources" (NCI) 349n
ginger 50, 152, 153
ginkgo biloba **148**, 153
ginseng
  diabetes mellitus 338
  drug interactions **148**
glandulars, defined **154**
glucosamine hydrochloride 152
Goodheart, George 106, **106**
Gram, Hans Burch 53
green tea research 152
guggul 46, 48, 49–50
guided imagery *see* imagery
gung, described 219

H

Hahnemann, Samuel Christian 35–36, 52–53
hand massage *see* massage therapy; reflexology
Harrington, Jane 141
Hartford Hospital, Web site address 381
Hatha yoga, described 228
headache
  biofeedback 193
  CAM therapies *11*
head cold, CAM therapies *11*
healers, traditional Native American medicine **80**
healing energy, crystals **248**
health care providers
  ayurvedic medicine 49
  CAM practitioners 15, 20–21, 23–28, **25**
  dietary supplements 146, 147
  probiotics 258
  reliable information 13–14
  risk prevention 17
  see also physicians; practitioners
health claims, regulation **356, 360–62**
health insurance *see* insurance coverage
heart disease, meditation **210–11**
heat therapy 128
  see also hydrotherapy
herbal supplements *see* botanical supplements; dietary supplements
HerbMed, Web site address 388

herbs
  defined **154**
  pain management 320
  traditional Chinese medicine 74–75
  traditional Native American medicine **80**
"Heritage and Health" (Indian Health Service) 79n
HHS *see* US Department of Health and Human Services
high blood pressure *see* hypertension
"History of Naturopathic Medicine" (American Association of Naturopathic Physicians) 59n
HIV *see* human immunodeficiency virus
homeo, defined 51
Home of Reflexology, Web site address 388
Homeopathic Pharmacopoeia of the United States, described 56
homeopathy
  defined **73, 116**
  described 35–36, 64
  like cures like **54**, 73
  overview 51–58
  vital force **52**
hospitals
  music therapy 313–14
  therapeutic touch **279**
hot compresses 128
Howell, Edward 249
"How Rolfing Works" (Rolf Institute of Structural Integration) 139n
human immunodeficiency virus (HIV), fraudulent claims 354–55
"Humor Therapy" (Wells) 297n
humor therapy, overview 297–300
Humphrey, Dana 79n
"Hydrotherapy" (WholeHealth Chicago) 125n
hydrotherapy, overview 125–29
hypertension (high blood pressure)
  aromatherapy 288
  meditation **210–11**
hypnos, defined 187
hypnosis
  dentistry **205**
  described 187, 190, **202**
  overview 201–5
  pain management 319

I

IBIDS Database *see* International Bibliographic Information on Dietary Supplements
ICAK-USA *see* International College of Applied Kinesiology-USA
ice therapy 127
imagery
    mental health 345
    overview 195–99
    relaxation 197
    see also hypnosis
incontinence, biofeedback 193
Indian Health Service, traditional Native American medicine publication 79n
"Information for the General Public" (American Society of Clinical Hypnosis) 201n
infusion, described 158
Ingham, Eunice **136**
insulin, defined **339**
insurance coverage
    acupuncture 99
    apitherapy 237
    CAM practitioners 24
    chiropractic 114–15
    light therapy 307
    massage therapists 132
    overview 365–74
    record keeping **367**
    Reiki 275
integration, Rolfing 141
integrative medicine, described 4
interconnectedness, ayurvedic medicine 41
International Bibliographic Information on Dietary Supplements (IBIDS Database), Web site address 389
International Center for Reiki Training
    contact information 386
    Reiki publication 269
    Web site address 380
International Chiropractors Association, contact information 386
International College of Applied Kinesiology-USA (ICAK-USA), applied kinesiology publication 105n

iron, vegetarianism 179–80
irritable bowel syndrome, traditional Chinese medicine 76
"Is a Vegetarian Diet Right for Me?" (Nemours Foundation) 177n
Iyangar yoga, described 228

J

Jaye, Vivian 141
Jiva Ayurveda, Web site address 389
Jnana yoga, described 228
joint pain, CAM therapies *11*
joke therapy *see* humor therapy

K

kapha, described 42, 43
Karma yoga, described 229
kava 162
Kellogg, J. H. 125
Kneipp, Sebastian 125
Krieger, Dolores 278
Kunz, Dora 278
Kushi, Aveline 169
Kushi, Michio 169

L

labels
    botanical supplements 162–63
    dietary supplements 147–48, **152**, **161**
    homeopathic remedies 55–56
lacto-ovo vegetarian, defined **178**
lacto vegetarian, defined **178**
laughter therapy *see* humor therapy
laxatives, defined **166**
laying on of hands, therapeutic touch **280**
legislation
    botanical supplements 157–58
    dietary supplements **47**
    ephedrine **150**
    homeopathic practitioners 55
    see also certification; regulation
libraries, reliable information 14
licensing *see* certification
lifestyles
    chelation therapy 241
    homeopathy 52, 53

lifestyles, continued
    naturopathic medicine 65
    traditional Native American
        medicine 80
light therapy
    defined 266
    overview 301–9
like cures like, homeopathy 52, 54, 73
lodestones 263
lordosis, Rolfing 140
low-back pain, chiropractic 111, 114,
    115–18

M

macrobiotic diet
    defined 178
    overview 169–71
    vegetarianism 178
"The Macrobiotic Diet" (Wong) 169n
magnesium, diabetes mellitus 338–39
magnetic therapy
    described 5
    overview 264–67
    pain management 320–27
"Magnetic Therapy" (Creighton
    University School of Medicine) 263n
magnets
    buying tips 326
    effectiveness 322
    health purposes 321
ma huang 151
Malhotra, Surender 211
"Manipulative and Body-Based Practices:
    An Overview" (NCCAM) 85n
manipulative therapy
    described 5, 89
    overview 85–90
    see also chiropractic medicine;
        osteopathic manipulation
mantra, described 212
"Massage Therapists" (DOL) 131n
massage therapy
    chiropractic 113
    defined 86
    mental health 345
    modalities 133
    overview 131–34
    pain management 319

massage therapy, continued
    Rolfing 142
    statistics 11, 85
    traditional Chinese medicine 74, 76
Mayo Foundation for Medical
    Education and Research, Web site
    address 379
McCall, Ray 142
McClain, Colleen 218
Medicinal Herb Garden, Web site
    address 389
meditation
    ayurvedic medicine 45
    described 187
    heart disease 210–11
    mental health 344
    overview 207–14
    statistics 11
    tai chi 224
    yoga 230
"Meditation for Health Purposes"
    (NCCAM) 207n
Medline Plus-Complementary and
    Alternative Therapies, Web site
    address 389
Memorial Sloan Kettering Cancer
    Center, Web site address 389
mental health care, alternative
    therapies 341–46
meridians
    defined 97
    described 32
Mesmer, Frank 264
meta-analysis, defined 116
metabolism, defined 252
mind-body medicine
    described 4
    disease treatment 190
    overview 185–90
    statistics 10
    see also biofeedback; cognitive
        behavioral therapy; hypnosis;
        relaxation therapy; spirituality
"Mind-Body Medicine" (A.D.A.M.,
    Inc.) 185n
mindfulness meditation 209
"Miracle Health Claims: Add a Dose of
    Skepticism" (FTC) 353n
modalities, described 133

movement therapy
  disease prevention **294**
  mental health 343
  tai chi 224
moxibustion
  described 32
  pain management 319
Mucuna pruriens 50
muscles
  Alexander technique 101–2
  applied kinesiology 105, 109
  Rolfing **140**
music therapy
  mental health 343
  overview 311–14
  research **312**
"Music Therapy Makes a Difference"
  (American Music Therapy
  Association) 311n
myofascial system, Rolfing 139

N

Nan Jing 71
National Association for Holistic
  Aromatherapy, contact
  information 386
National Ayurvedic Medical
  Association, contact information 386
National Cancer Institute (NCI)
  Office of Cancer Complementary
    and Alternative Medicine,
    contact information 387
  publications
    cancer treatments 329n
    health information 349n
  Web site address 380
National Center for Complementary
  and Alternative Medicine
  (NCCAM)
  contact information 386
  publications
    acupuncture 95n
    ayurvedic medicine 39n
    CAM practitioners 23n
    cancer treatment 329n
    chiropractic medicine 111n
    complementary and alternative
      medicine 3n, 13n

National Center for Complementary
  and Alternative Medicine
  (NCCAM), continued
  publications, continued
    dietary supplements 145n
    financial issues 365n
    homeopathy 51n
    magnets, pain management 317n
    manipulative and body-based
      practices 85n
    meditation 207n
    prayer 215n
    spirituality 215n
    US complementary and
      alternative medicine 7n
    whole medical systems 31n
National Center for Homeopathy,
  Web site address 381
National Certification Commission
  for Acupuncture and Oriental
  Medicine, contact information 387
National Institute of Ayurvedic
  Medicine, contact information 387
National Institute of Diabetes and
  Digestive and Kidney Diseases
  (NIDDK), diabetes treatment
  publication 337n
National Institute of Environmental
  Health Sciences, Web site
  address 379
National Institutes of Health
  (NIH) botanical supplements
  publication 157n
  Office of Dietary Supplements,
    contact information 387
National Pain Foundation, Web site
  address 381
National Qigong Association
  contact information 387
  qigong publication 219n
Native American medicine
  see traditional Native American
  medicine
natural products
  described 15
  statistics *11*
naturopathic doctors (ND)
  defined **60**
  treatment modalities **64**

naturopathic medicine (naturopathy)
  defined **58, 73, 116–17**
  described 34–35
  disease 35
  overview 59–65
NCCAM *see* National Center for
  Complementary and Alternative
  Medicine
NCI *see* National Cancer Institute
ND *see* naturopathic doctors
needles *see* acupuncture
Nei Jing 71
Nemours Foundation
  publications
    detox diets 165n
    vegetarian diets 177n
  Web site address 380, 381
nerve flow, chiropractic 112
neurotransmitters, acupuncture 33, 99
NIDDK *see* National Institute of Diabetes
  and Digestive and Kidney Diseases
NOAH-Complementary and Alternative
  Medicine, Web site address 389
Nolte, Dorothy 141
Norris, Patricia 197
nurses, therapeutic touch **279**
nutrition *see* diet and nutrition
nutritional supplements *see* dietary
  supplements

O

obesity, pediatric blood pressure **211**
observational study, defined **117**
Ohlgren, Gael 141
Ohsawa, George 169
Oriental medicine, described 64
orthopedist, defined **117**
osteopathic manipulation, defined **86**
"Osteopathic Medicine" (American
  Association of Colleges of
  Osteopathic Medicine) 67n
osteopathic medicine (osteopathy)
  defined **73, 117**
  overview 67–69
osteoporosis, defined **117**
Otikon Otic Solution 35
otitis media, research 35
ovo vegetarian, defined **178**

P

pain management
  acupressure 93–94
  acupuncture 32–33, 98
  Alexander technique 103
  CAM therapies *11*
  dependencies **320**
  hydrotherapy 127
  otitis media 35
  overview 317–27
  therapeutic touch 278
Palmer, Daniel David 109, 111–12, 265
panchakarma, described 44–45
pancreas, defined **339**
parasympathetic nervous system,
  described 212
pastoral counseling, mental health 342
pathos, defined 51
Perkins, Elisha 263
pesci vegetarian, defined **178**
"Philosophy" (American Association of
  Naturopathic Physicians) 59n
physiatric techniques, pain
  management 318–19
physical medicine, described 64
physicians
  alternative medicine **18–19**
  naturopathic medicine 60
  osteopathy 67–69
  see also practitioners
phytochemicals 174
phytoestrogens 169–70
piezoelectric effect 244, 248
Pinellia **151**
pitta, described 42, 43
placebo, defined **58, 97, 117**
postural analysis, applied kinesiology 108
potentization, described 53
power yoga, described 228
"Practice Modalities" (American
  Association of Naturopathic
  Physicians) 59n
practitioners
  acupressure 94
  acupuncture 99
  apitherapy 236
  ayurvedic medicine 46–47
  biofeedback 194

practitioners, continued
  complementary and alternative
    medicine 15, 20–21
  guided imagery 199
  hydrotherapy 129
  hypnosis 203–4
  music therapy 312–13
  naturopathic medicine
    59–60, **60**
  reflexology 137
  Reiki 270–71
  selection process 23–28
  therapeutic touch 281
  traditional Chinese medicine
    74–75, 77
  see also physicians
prakriti 42
praxis, defined 111
prayer
  described **216**
  overview 215–18
  statistics *11*
  studies 9–10
"Prayer and Spirituality in Health:
  Ancient Practices, Modern
  Science" (NCCAM) 215n
preclinical study, defined **97**
pregnancy
  acupressure 94
  aromatherapy 287
  botanical supplements **160**
  enzyme therapy 253
  hydrotherapy 129
  massage therapy 132
  Reiki 273
  yoga 232
Priessnitz, Vincenz 125
primary control, Alexander
  technique 102
principle of similars 36
probiotics
  overview 255–62
  selection guidelines **261**
progressive muscle relaxation,
  described 187
propolis
  defined **236**
  research 35
proteins, vegetarianism 180

psychotherapy
  hypnosis 204–5
  magnetic therapy 266–67
pulsed field therapy, described 5

Q

qi
  acupressure 92
  defined **97**
  described 32, 71
  qigong 219
  tai chi 223, 224
  therapeutic touch 277
  traditional Chinese medicine 76
qigong
  defined **73**
  overview 219–21
  traditional Chinese medicine 71, 74
Qigong Institute, contact
  information 387
Quackwatch, Web site address 389
quartz, described 244, 246
"Questions and Answers About Cancer
  And Complementary And Alternative
  Medicine" (NCCAM) 329n
"Questions and Answers About
  Chelation Therapy" (American
  Heart Association) 239n
"Questions and Answers About
  Homeopathy" (NCCAM) 51n
"Questions and Answers about Seasonal
  Affective Disorder and Light Therapy"
  (Society for Light Treatment and
  Biological Rhythms) 301n
"Questions and Answers About
  Using Magnets To Treat Pain"
  (NCCAM) 317n

R

radio psychiatry, mental health 346
Raja yoga, described 229
raw food diet
  overview 173–76
  side effects **174**
"The Raw Food Diet" (Wong) 173n
Raynaud's disease, biofeedback 193
referrals, CAM practitioners 23–24

reflexology
  defined 86
  described 93
  history 136
  overview 135–38
Reflexology Association of America,
  contact information 388
refractory, defined 266
regulation
  acupuncture needles 96
  botanical supplements 157–58
  dietary supplements 15, 148–49, 356,
    360–62
  fraudulent claims 363
  health claims 356, 360–62
  herbal remedies 78
  homeopathy 55–56
  TCM practitioners 77
  see also certification; legislation
Reiki, overview 269–75
"Reiki, Questions and Answers"
  (International Center for Reiki
  Training) 269
relaxation response, described 188–89
relaxation therapy, described 186–87, 190
remedies
  described 51–52, 55
  regulation 55–56
Reston, James 72
risks
  CAM therapies 17, 26–27
  manipulative therapies 88–89
Rolf, Ida P. 139, 141, 142
Rolfing
  defined 86
  overview 139–42
"Rolfing and Massage" (Rolf Institute of
  Structural Integration) 139n
"Rolfing Structural Integration" (Rolf
  Institute of Structural Integration) 139n
Rolf Institute of Structural Integration
  contact information 388
  Rolfing publication 139n
"Rolf Movement" (Rolf Institute of
  Structural Integration) 139n
Rosenfeld, Barry 218
Rossman, Martin L. 195–96
royal jelly, defined 236
ruby, described 247

S

SAD see seasonal affective disorder
safety concerns
  acupuncture 96
  ayurvedic medicine 48
  botanical supplements 160–61, 162–63
  colonic irrigation 126
  complementary and alternative
    medicine 13–21
  detox diets 165, 167–68
  dietary supplements 148, 154–55
  fraudulent claims 356–57
  hydrotherapy 129
  macrobiotic diet 171
  probiotics 258
  raw food diet 175–76
  St. John's wort 148
  Web site information 14
  yoga 231–32
St. John's wort
  AIDS therapy 356–57
  drug interactions 148
SAMHSA see Substance Abuse and
  Mental Health Services Administration
Sanfeng, Zhang 223
sapphire, described 247
seasonal affective disorder (SAD),
  light therapy 301–9
"Selecting a Complementary and
  Alternative Medicine (CAM)
  Practitioner" (NCCAM) 23n
self-help, mental health 341–42
semi-vegetarian, defined 178
sham, defined 117
shiatsu 93
Sida cordifolia 151
side effects
  CAM therapies 26
  chiropractic 114
  enzyme therapy 253
  homeopathic remedies 56–57
  humor therapy 299
  light therapy 305
  macrobiotic diet 171
  magnetic therapy 325–26
  raw food diets 174
  therapeutic touch 280–81
  similia principle 52

sitz baths 128
Society for Light Treatment and
   Biological Rhythms
   contact information 388
   seasonal affective disorder
      publication 301n
Solomon, George 185
soy research 152
Spiegel, David 187–88
spinal manipulation
   see chiropractic medicine
spirituality
   cancer treatment 333–36
   described 187, 190, 216
   overview 215–18
"Spirituality in Cancer Care"
   (NCI) 329n
Starsong, Heather 141
statistics
   acupuncture 95–96
   ayurvedic medicine 40, 41
   CAM therapies 7–12, 85
   chiropractic 112
   dance therapy 293–94
   homeopathy 54
   osteopathic physicians 68
   prayer 215–16
Still, Andrew Taylor 67
stomach upset, CAM therapies 11
Stoney, Catherine 216
stress management
   acupressure 93
   mind-body medicine 188
   naturopathic medicine 65
   reflexology 136
   Rolfing 139
structural integration see Rolfing
structure, applied kinesiology 108, 109
subluxation, chiropractic 112
Substance Abuse and Mental Health
   Services Administration (SAMHSA),
   mental health care publication 341n
supplements see botanical supplements;
   dietary supplements
surgical procedures
   hypnosis 204
   naturopathic medicine 65
Susruta Samhita 40
Sutherland, William 123

sympathetic nervous system, described 212
systematic review, defined 117

T

tai chi
   described 71, 76
   overview 223–26
"Tai Chi" (A.D.A.M., Inc.) 223n
Tantra yoga, described 229
technology, mental health
   treatments 345–46
telemedicine, mental health 345
telephone counseling, mental
   health 345–46
Ten Series, Rolfing 140
Thatcher, C. J. 265
"Therapeutic Touch" (A.D.A.M.,
   Inc.) 277n
therapeutic touch, overview 277–81
thermal biofeedback, described 191
Thunder God vine 34
tinctures, described 158
"Tips for the Savvy Supplement
   User" (FDA) 145n
tobacco use, complementary and
   alternative medicine 9
toxicology, defined 58
toxins
   defined 166
   described 165
traditional Chinese medicine (TCM)
   defined 97
   described 31–32
   mental health 343–44
   overview 71–78
"Traditional Chinese Medicine"
   (WholeHealth Chicago) 71n
traditional Native American medicine
   mental health 344
   overview 79–81
training see certification
trance, described 201
transcendental meditation,
   described 209–12
Treiber, Frank 211
triad of health, applied kinesiology 106,
   109–10
Tripterygium wilfordii Hook F 34

Tsevat, Joel 217
tuina 76, 93
turmeric 46, 50, 152
type 1 diabetes, defined **339**
type 2 diabetes, defined **339**

U

University of Washington, Web site
    address 389
Upledger, John E. 123–24
Upledger Institute, Inc., craniosacral
    therapy publication 121n
urinary tract infections (UTI),
    cranberries 35
US Department of Health and Human
    Services (DHHS; HHS), Web site
    address 380
US Department of Labor (DOL),
    massage therapy publication 131n
"The Use of Complementary and
    Alternative Medicine in the United
    States" (NCCAM) 7n
US Federal Trade Commission (FTC)
    complaint information 359, 363
    health claim regulations **356, 360–62**
    miracle health claims publication 353n
    safety considerations 16
US Food and Drug Administration (FDA)
    contact information 388
    dietary supplement safety 15, 16
    dietary supplements publication 145n

V

valerian 162, 320
vanadium, diabetes mellitus 339–40
vata, described 42, 43
veda, defined 39
vegan, defined **178**
vegetarian diets, overview 177–82
vegetarians
    described **178**
    food variety **182**
visualization
    mental health 345
    overview 195–99
    pain management 318
vital energy *see* qi

vital points therapy 45
vitamin B12, vegetarianism 180
vitamin C, research 35
vitamin D, vegetarianism 180

W

Wasserman, Michael R. 298
water therapy *see* hydrotherapy
Wells, Ken R. 297n
"What Is Applied Kinesiology"
    (ICAK-USA) 105n
"What is Ayurvedic Medicine"
    (NCCAM) 39n
"What Is Complementary and
    Alternative Medicine (CAM)?"
    (NCCAM) 3n
"What Is Naturopathic Medicine?"
    (American Association of
    Naturopathic Physicians) 59n
"What is Qigong?" (National Qigong
    Association) 219n
"What's in the Bottle? An Introduction to
    Dietary Supplements" (NCCAM) 145n
"When Worlds Collide" (Humphrey) 79n
WholeHealth Chicago
    publications
        acupressure 91n
        Alexander technique 101n
        hydrotherapy 125n
        traditional Chinese medicine 71n
    Web site address 379
whole medical systems
    described 4
    overview 31–37
    see also acupuncture; ayurvedic medicine;
        homeopathy; naturopathic medicine;
        traditional Chinese medicine
"Whole Medical Systems: An Overview"
    (NCCAM) 31n
Wong, Cathy 169n, 173n

Y

yang
    acupuncture 98
    described 31–32, **33**
    traditional Chinese medicine 72
    see also yin

yin
  acupuncture 98
  described 31–32, **33**
  traditional Chinese
    medicine 72
  see also yang
yoga
  ayurvedic medicine 45
  described **231**
  mental health 344

yoga, continued
  overview 227–32
  statistics *11*
  "Yoga" (A.D.A.M., Inc.) 227n

Z

zinc
  dietary supplements 146
  vegetarianism 180